Praise for *Johns Hopkins Evidence-Based Practice: Implementation and Translation*

*"From the bedside to the boardroom, the Johns Hop~.
for the translation of new knowledge into practice and eviden~.
The model transcends the professions and provides structure and rigo~ ~
decision making in a complex environment."*

Deb Zimmermann, DNP, RN, NEA-BC
Chief Nursing Officer and Vice President, Patient Care Services
VCU Health System

*"We applaud you and the authors. We have adopted the model at Virginia
Commonwealth University Health System, and the text is used to teach our
1,000+ nursing students evidence-based practice in our school of nursing."*

Diane Pravikoff, RN, PhD, FAAN
Director of Research/Professional Liaison
CINAHL Information Systems

*"Implementation of evidence-based practice in nursing is not a simple process.
It requires both individual and organizational commitment, along with a great
deal of preparation, knowledge, and skill. The authors have presented essential
information from their own experiences to guide readers through this process.
They describe the infrastructure, core competencies, and skills necessary to manage evidence-based practice projects, to achieve meaningful clinical outcomes,
and, equally important, disseminate the results.* Johns Hopkins Evidence-Based
Practice Model: Implementation and Translation *combines the theoretical with the
practical and will be extremely helpful to individuals at any stage of implementing evidence-based practice in various health care settings."*

Linda P. Riley, PhD, RN
Director, Nursing Research and Evidence Based Practice
Children's Health care of Atlanta

"This book provides invaluable information to facilitate the growth of evidence-based practice at the bedside and across the health care system. Johns Hopkins Nursing Evidence-Based Practice Model: Implementation and Translation *provides much needed guidance to avoid the pitfalls often encountered during successful translation of evidence to practice."*

Nancy Dunton, PhD
Associate Research Professor
University of Kansas Medical Center

JOHNS HOPKINS NURSING
EVIDENCE-BASED PRACTICE
IMPLEMENTATION AND TRANSLATION

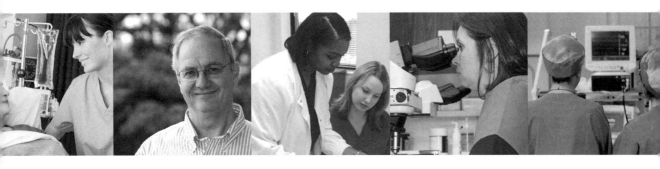

Edited by
Stephanie S. Poe, DNP, RN, and
Kathleen M. White, PhD, RN, NEA-BC, FAAN

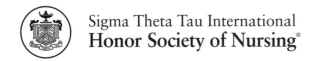

Sigma Theta Tau International
Honor Society of Nursing®

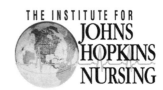

THE INSTITUTE FOR
JOHNS
HOPKINS
NURSING

Sigma Theta Tau International

Sigma Theta Tau International
550 West North Street
Indianapolis, IN 46202

To order additional books, buy in bulk, or order for corporate use, contact Nursing Knowledge International at 888.NKI.4YOU (888.654.4968/US and Canada) or +1.317.634.8171 (outside US and Canada).

To request a review copy for course adoption, e-mail solutions@nursingknowledge.org or call 888.NKI.4YOU (888.654.4968/US and Canada) or +1.317.917.4983 (outside US and Canada).

To request author information, or for speaker or other media requests, contact Rachael McLaughlin of the Honor Society of Nursing, Sigma Theta Tau International at 888.634.7575 (US and Canada) or +1.317.634.8171 (outside US and Canada).

ISBN-13: 978-1-930538-85-6

Library of Congress Cataloging-in-Publication Data

Poe, Stephanie.

 Johns Hopkins nursing evidence-based practice : implementation and translation / Stephanie Poe and Kathleen White.

 p. ; cm.

 Other title: Nursing evidence-based practice

 Includes bibliographical references.

 ISBN 978-1-930538-91-7

 1. Evidence-based nursing. I. White, Kathleen M., 1940- II. Sigma Theta Tau International. III. Johns Hopkins University. IV. Title. V. Title: Nursing evidence-based practice.

 [DNLM: 1. Evidence-Based Nursing--organization & administration. 2. Clinical Competence. 3. Leadership. 4. Translational Research. WY 100.7 P743j 2010]

 RT42.P65 2010

 610.73--dc22

 2010019437

Publisher: Renee Wilmeth	**Development Editor:** Bill Kelly
Acquisitions Editors: Cynthia Saver, MS, RN, and Janet Boivin, RN	**Principal Editor:** Carla Hall
Editorial Coordinator: Paula Jeffers	**Copy Editor:** Kevin Kent
Proofreaders: Billy Fields and Barbara Bennett	**Indexer:** Johnna VanHoose Dinse
Cover Design, Interior Design, and Page Composition: Louisa Adair, Studio Galou	

First Printing, 2010

Dedication

This book is dedicated to the nurses and nursing students who embrace evidence-based professional practice. This transformational change is not possible without visionary nurse leaders who strive to create a learning environment distinguished by spirited inquiry and innovation.

Acknowledgements

The editors would like to acknowledge Jane Shivnan, MScN, RN, AOCN, executive director of the The Institute for Johns Hopkins Nursing, for her assistance with final review and editing of the manuscript.

SP would like to acknowledge her family whose unwavering love and support have enabled her to pursue this vision.

KW would like to acknowledge the love and support from her husband and sons who have always encouraged her to follow her professional endeavors.

About the Editors

Stephanie S. Poe, DNP, RN

Stephanie Poe is director of nursing, clinical quality, and chief nursing information officer at The Johns Hopkins Hospital, Baltimore, Maryland, USA, where she holds a joint appointment with The Johns Hopkins University School of Nursing. She is a respected author and speaker on a wide variety of interdisciplinary quality, safety, informatics, and evidence-based practice topics. Poe was one of the original developers of the Johns Hopkins Nursing Evidence-Based Practice (JHNEBP) Model. She has extensive experience developing EBP competencies in nurse leaders and bedside nurses, and guiding clinical information system design to embed evidence-based nursing practices into clinical work flow.

Kathleen M. White, PhD, RN, NEA-BC, FAAN

Kathleen White is associate professor and director of the Doctor of Nursing Practice Program at The Johns Hopkins University School of Nursing (JHUSON), Baltimore, Maryland, USA. She holds a joint appointment as a clinical nurse specialist at The Johns Hopkins Hospital (JHH) and as nurse research liaison at Howard County General Hospital. She is a member of a collaborative team of JHH and JHUSON staff that developed the Johns Hopkins Nursing Evidence-Based Practice (JHNEBP) Model and Guidelines. This model has been highlighted in several publications, including the *Journal of Nursing Administration* and the *Advisory Board Practice Exemplar* series. The research conducted on the JHNEBP model won the 2005 Sigma Theta Tau International Research Utilization Award. White has been an active participant in many quality and safety initiatives and has received numerous practice grants. In 2007 she was appointed chair of the Maryland Patient Safety Center's board of directors.

About the Contributing Authors

Chapter 1: Transforming Nursing Practice Through Evidence

Sandra L. Dearholt, MS, RN

Sandra Dearholt is currently the assistant director of nursing for neurosciences and psychiatry at The Johns Hopkins Hospital, Baltimore, Maryland, USA. She has an extensive clinical background in critical care, nursing administration, and staff development. Dearholt has written a variety of articles on evidence-based practice and has spoken extensively on the topic. Her special areas of interest are the development of strategies for incorporating evidence into practice at the bedside, fostering professional practice standards, and service excellence through patient-centered care. Dearholt is also a co-author of *Johns Hopkins Nursing Evidence-Based Practice Model and Guidelines* (2007).

Sidebar Authors

Transforming Outpatient Nursing Practice Through Evidence

Julie Kubiak, RN, MS, PCRN
Assistant Director of Nursing for Ambulatory Care
The Johns Hopkins Hospital
Baltimore, Maryland, USA

Mary A. Rice, MBA, MSN
Director of Nursing for Ambulatory Care
The Johns Hopkins Hospital
Baltimore, Maryland, USA

Chapter 2: Assessing Leadership Readiness

Deborah Dang, PhD, RN, NEA-BC

Deborah Dang is the director of nursing, practice, education, and research at The Johns Hopkins Hospital, Baltimore, Maryland, USA, and holds a joint appointment with The Johns Hopkins University School of Nursing. For the past 10 years, she has guided the transformation of the nursing culture at The Johns Hopkins Hospital to one of practice based on evidence. She has consulted and presented regionally and nationally on the topic of evidence-based practice. She is an active health services researcher who studies structural and process factors in the nursing practice environment that impact patient outcomes, and was the recipient of the 2006 AcademyHealth Interdisciplinary Research Group on Nursing Issues New Investigator Award. She is committed to creating and sustaining practice environments that foster nurses' roles in improving patient outcomes. Dang has served on statewide workgroups and has a longstanding interest in organizational change: She led major efforts at Hopkins, including a multiyear imple-mentation of a hospital-wide redesign of the Patient Care Delivery Model, development and implementation of a nursing salaried compensation model, and creation of the ideal medication-use system to guide new building planning.

Stephanie S. Poe, DNP, RN

See Stephanie Poe's bio on page vii.

Sidebar Author

Lessons Learned: Transformational Leadership in a Community Hospital Setting

Larry Strassner, PhD, RN, NEA-BC
Vice President for Nursing and Chief Nursing Officer
Franklin Square Hospital
Baltimore, Maryland, USA

Chapter 3: Establishing Organizational Infrastructure

Robin Newhouse, PhD, RN, NEA-BC

Robin Newhouse is associate professor and assistant dean for the Doctor of Nursing Practice Program at the University of Maryland School of Nursing, Baltimore, Mary-land, USA. She has published, presented, and consulted nationally and internationally on the topic of evidence-based nursing practice. Newhouse was the first author on the *Johns Hopkins Nursing Evidence-Based Practice Model and Guidelines*, published in 2007 by the Honor Society of Nursing, Sigma Theta Tau International (STTI). Her areas of expertise include evidence-based practice, health services research methods, study of health care processes and related outcomes, and quality of care. As a health services researcher, her funded studies focus on application of research to practice and patient outcomes. Newhouse is a member of the American Nurses Credentialing Cen-ter's Research Council, is chair of the Research and Scholarship Council for STTI, and is an invited member of the Advisory Council in Evidence-Based Behavioral Practice at Northwestern University, as a representative for nursing.

Chapter 4: Building Core Competencies in Nursing Service

Stephanie S. Poe, DNP, RN

See Stephanie Poe's bio on page vii.

Sidebar Authors

Neuroscience Academy

Sandra L. Dearholt, MS, RN
See Sandra Dearholt's bio on page viii.

Barbara Fitzsimons, MS, RN, CNRN
Nurse Educator, Department of Neurosciences
The Johns Hopkins Hospital
Baltimore, Maryland, USA

Building Competencies Through an EBP Fellowship

Sue Verrillo, MSN, RN
Nurse Manager, Department of Rehabilitation Medicine
The Johns Hopkins Hospital
Baltimore, Maryland, USA

Chapter 5: Building Core Competencies in Nursing Academia

Sarah J. McDermott Shaefer, RN, PhD

Sarah Shaefer is an assistant professor, the coordinator of the course The Research Process in Nursing at The Johns Hopkins University School of Nursing, Baltimore, Maryland, USA, and the chair of the Baccalaureate Curriculum Committee. She is a member of The Johns Hopkins Nursing Evidence-Based Practice (JHNEBP) Steering Committee. She has significant experience in teaching EBP to clinical nurse leaders as well as bedside and student nurses. Shaefer significantly expanded collaboration between bedside and student nurses on current EBP projects. She has presented data on student satisfaction with these collaborations internationally. She teaches and mentors clinicians and students on the EBP process. Her research focus is excellence in teaching and learning.

Kathleen M. White, PhD, RN, NEA-BC, FAAN

See Kathleen White's bio on page vii.

Sidebar Authors

EBP & Pediatric Rehabilitation

Elizabeth DiPietro, MS, RN
Clinical Specialist
Kennedy Krieger Institute
Baltimore, Maryland, USA

Tami W. Swearingen, RN, BS, MA, LNCC
Senior Vice President of Nursing and Patient Services
Kennedy Krieger Institute
Baltimore, Maryland, USA

Sarah J. M. Shaefer, PhD, RN
See Sarah Shaefer's bio listed previously on this page.

Chapter 6: Managing the EBP Project

Stephanie S. Poe, DNP, RN

See Stephanie Poe's bio on page vii.

Patricia B. Dawson, MSN, RN

Patricia Dawson is the assistant director of nursing clinical quality and Magnet at The Johns Hopkins Hospital, Baltimore, Maryland, USA. She has experience in working with nurses at all levels to identify, develop, and disseminate best practices in clinical care and leadership that are worthy of Magnet recognition. She facilitates the implementation of evidence-based guidelines in the practice setting and instructs nurses on conduct of clinical outcome measurement. Dawson has presented and published on diverse topics related to quality improvement and patient safety.

Sidebar Author

Distractions and Interruptions to Medication Administration

Annette L. Perschke, DNP, RN, CRRN
Project Leader, Clinical Quality and Informatics
The Johns Hopkins Hospital
Baltimore, Maryland, USA

Chapter 7: Outcomes and Evaluation

Kathleen White, PhD, RN, NEA-BC, FAAN

See Kathleen White's bio on page vii.

Chapter 8: Selecting the Pathway to Translation

Maria Cvach, MS, RN, CCRN

Maria Cvach is assistant director of nursing, clinical standards, at The Johns Hopkins Hospital, Baltimore, Maryland, USA. She is chair of the Evidence-Based Practice Steering Committee at The Johns Hopkins Hospital and coordinates the internal EBP workshops for staff. Cvach supervises The Johns Hopkins Hospital EBP fellow and facilitates and monitors EBP projects performed by The Johns Hopkins Hospital Nursing Standards of Care Committee. She has conducted numerous EBP projects on various topics, such as cardiac monitor alarm management, fall injury prediction, medication double-checks, sedation assessment tools, and shift fatigue. Cvach works closely with The Johns Hopkins University School of Nursing students on EBP projects selected by the hospital. She has written on a variety of topics, such as fall prediction and assessment tools, and various cardiac issues, including monitor-alarm fatigue and complex cardiac drugs.

Mei Ching Lee, MS, RN

Mei Ching Lee is a nurse research associate for the department of nursing at The Johns Hopkins Hospital, Baltimore, Maryland, USA. She is a PhD candidate in nursing and has more than 20 years of clinical experience. Lee gained considerable EBP knowledge, skills, and expertise as a department of nursing EBP fellow. She has spoken on topics related to EBP, chaired a unit-based EBP committee, conducted successful EBP projects, and coordinated EBP workshops for staff nurses.

Sidebar Authors

Selection of a Sedation Scale

Laura Kress, RN, MAS
Assistant Director of Nursing, Professional Practice
The Johns Hopkins Hospital
Baltimore, Maryland, USA

Medication Safety: To Check or Not to Check

Maria Cvach, MS, RN, CCRN
See Maria Cvach's bio on page xi.

Mei Ching Lee, MS, RN
See Mei Ching Lee's bio listed previously on this page.

Translating Safe Sleep Evidence Into Nursing Practice

Sarah J. M. Shaefer, PhD, RN
See Sarah Shaefer's bio on page x.

Sandra J. Frank, JD, CAE
Executive Director
Tomorrow's Child/Michigan SIDS
Lansing, Michigan, USA

Mary Adkins, BA, MSW
Program Director
Tomorrow's Child/Michigan SIDS
Lansing, Michigan, USA

Mary Terhaar, DNSc, RN
Assistant Professor
Department of Health Systems and Outcomes
The Johns Hopkins University School of Nursing
Baltimore, Maryland, USA

Chapter 9: Applying Translation Science to Improve Health Outcomes

Linda L. Costa, PhD, RN, NEA-BC

Linda Costa is the nurse researcher at The Johns Hopkins Hospital, Baltimore, Maryland, USA. She holds a joint appointment at The Johns Hopkins University School of Nursing, where she teaches in the health systems management track of the master's program. She has extensive experience mentoring nurse leaders in evidence-based practice and development of research studies. Costa's research focus is on medication safety and medication management. She holds a certification in Nursing Case Management from American Nurses Credentialing Center (ANCC) and is a member of the Nursing Research Review Committee of the American Nurses Foundation.

Terry Nelson, MSN, RN

Terry Nelson is assistant director of medical nursing at The Johns Hopkins Hospital, Baltimore, Maryland, USA. She has held a variety of leadership positions and has broad experience in management, quality improvement, safety, efficiency, regulatory standards, and disaster management. Nelson has written about and spoken on topics of quality improvement, core measures, rapid response team implementation, disaster preparation, and pain management. She holds memberships in Sigma Theta Tau International, American Organization of Nurse Executives, and Phi Kappa Phi.

Chapter 10: Translating and Sharing Results

Kathleen White, PhD, RN, NEA-BC, FAAN

See Kathleen White's bio on page vii.

Foreword

Once again, it is our pleasure to bring you the latest Johns Hopkins Nursing publication, *Johns Hopkins Nursing Evidence-Based Practice: Implementation and Translation.* Stephanie Poe and Kathleen White, two of the original developers of the Johns Hopkins Nursing Evidence-Based Practice Model and Guidelines, edited this book, and they have included many other Johns Hopkins nurses as authors of chapters and vignettes in order to share what we have learned as we continue to refine our model.

Three years ago, Sigma Theta Tau published *Johns Hopkins Nursing Evidence-Based Practice Model and Guidelines,* which was also written by a team of nurse leaders and faculty from The Johns Hopkins Hospital and The Johns Hopkins University School of Nursing. The book enjoyed tremendous success, was listed as one of the top 10 selling books from Nursing Knowledge International for 2008, and was praised by reviewers for presenting a practical and user-friendly approach to evidence-based practice (EBP). It focused on the development of the Johns Hopkins Nursing EBP model and presented step-by-step guidelines for planning and developing an EBP program.

Since that publication, Johns Hopkins Nursing has continued to focus on developing evidence-based practice, creating a culture of critical thinking and ongoing learning for both students and nursing staff, and fostering a professional environment where evidence supports clinical, educational, and administrative decision making. Nonetheless, numerous barriers to EBP integration by nurses remain in clinical settings. Our experience has proven the importance of planning the implementation of EBP as a strategic initiative and developing a systematic approach to translating evidence into practice. These strategies and the development of successful partnerships between the hospital and the school of nursing, and between the nursing services and hospital administration, are critical for teaching, using, and sustaining EBP.

Johns Hopkins Nursing Evidence-Based Practice: Implementation and Translation provides additional advice on meeting the complex challenges associated with EBP implementation and translation. The authors have included numerous practical examples that illustrate key considerations in implementing EBP and translating findings into practice. The book includes a helpful discussion of important steps, including

- Leadership and planning for EBP

- Identification, measurement, monitoring and evaluation of outcomes

- Translation techniques

- Dissemination techniques

We hope you enjoy this book and the value it can add to your EBP.

Karen Haller, PhD, RN, FAAN
Vice President for Nursing and Patient Care Serivces, Chief Nursing Officer
The Johns Hopkins Hospital
Baltimore, Maryland

Martha N. Hill, PhD, RN, FAAN
Dean, The Johns Hopkins University School of Nursing
Baltimore, Maryland

Introduction

Johns Hopkins Nursing Evidence-Based Practice: Implementation and Translation is dedicated to identifying methods to successfully implement evidence-based practice (EBP) in organizations and translate evidence-based findings into practice. This book is an extension of our previous work, which introduced the model and guidelines and armed readers with tools to plan and develop an EBP program. The goal of the current book is to share information and a pathway to follow when managing the structure, process, and outcomes of EBP projects and translating evidence in a variety of health care settings. The three sections of this book provide practical guidelines for implementation and translation of evidence to achieve excellence in professional practice and quality patient outcomes.

Section I discusses the infrastructure components of establishing an evidence-based environment. Chapter 1 provides a brief overview of the Johns Hopkins Nursing Evidence-Based Practice (JHNEBP) Model, identifying linkages with the American Nurses Credentialing Center's Magnet Recognition Program. Chapter 2 focuses on creating a road map for assessment of the organization's leadership team and capacity to adopt EBP. Chapter 3 presents strategies to integrate EBP into the organizational culture and to establish critical infrastructure.

Section II lays out the strategies to build capacity for translation. Chapter 4 centers on the preparation of nurses for EBP leadership through staff development. Chapter 5 considers the preparation of students for professional practice and the integration of EBP into school of nursing curricula. Chapter 6 offers strategies for successful EBP project management. Chapter 7 provides information on how to measure and analyze EBP outcomes.

Section III is devoted to translation. Chapter 8 explores factors to consider in choosing the appropriate translation strategy. Chapter 9 provides a method to assess organizational readiness to adopt a new practice within the context of the external environment and the internal practice milieu. Finally, Chapter 10 discusses the important role of dissemination of outcomes of EBP initiatives.

Johns Hopkins Nursing Evidence-Based Practice: Implementation and Translation is a collaborative work between The Johns Hopkins Hospital and The Johns Hopkins University School of Nursing. It allows the reader to benefit from the depth and breadth of experience of a long-term collaboration among nurse leaders in service and academic settings in their quest to achieve exemplary nursing practice.

Contents

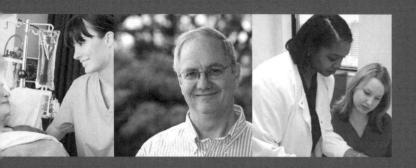

PART I

Transforming Nursing Practice
Through Evidence

Evidence-based practice (EBP) is an explicit process that enables clinicians to seek out best practices and make determinations regarding if and how these practices can be incorporated into patient care. Clinicians practicing EBP seek out the best available evidence to inform decisions to provide the highest quality and most effective care for patients (Wolff & Desch, 2005). The ultimate goal of this process is the improvement of patient care outcomes.

This chapter explores the rapidly growing demand for health care and nursing organizations to create cultures that foster the use of EBP to support decision making and to meet the challenges that result from this transformation. To achieve excellence and innovation in patient care through EBP, the organization must first adopt a working EBP model. The organization must then empower staff and provide the resources and support to enable clinicians to effectively translate EBP findings into everyday practice.

The Need to Implement EBP

In today's health care environment, many factors call for an EBP approach to the provision of care—for example, health care consumers exert increasing demand for higher quality health care, third-party payers require evidence-based interventions, continual efforts are needed to contain costs, and new pay-for-performance reimbursement structures exist. The groundbreaking Institute of Medicine (IOM) report, *Crossing the Quality Chasm* (2001, p. 2), points out that "medical science and technology have advanced at a rapid pace; however, the health care delivery system has floundered in its ability to provide consistently high-quality care to all Americans. Research on the quality of care reveals a health care system that frequently falls short in its ability to translate knowledge into practice, and to apply new technology safely and appropriately." Wolf and Greenhouse (2007) identified five trends that reinforce the need to use an evidence-based approach to practice in developing effective care delivery systems for the future:

1. Changes in patients' level of knowledge

2. Changes in the types of clinicians and settings needed

3. Advances in medicine

4. Advances in information technology (IT)

5. Changes in reimbursement

Changes in Patients' Level of Knowledge

Many patients are now better informed about their conditions and available treatments than they have been in the past. They have easy access through the Internet to the most recent medical research and databases around the world. Patients can also exchange information with large numbers of other patients experiencing the same condition through listservs, chat lines, and global social-networking websites. They can share information about institutions, doctors, and treatment plans. As a result, patients often expect more of health care providers and tolerate less. They are well aware of the flaws and broken systems in health care, such as the high rate of medication errors, and they drive necessary reform by insisting that deficiencies be corrected. Future care delivery systems need to find effective ways to "include patients as partners and to capitalize on [the patients'] knowledge" (Wolf & Greenhouse, 2007, p. 383). An EBP approach can help organizations identify effective strategies for using the Internet to provide accurate information to patients and can enable the development of new online forums, such as professionally guided support groups or patient focus groups providing health care organizations with feedback regarding their patient-care experiences.

Changes in Types of Clinicians and Settings Needed

Because of the ongoing trend to discharge patients sooner and to transition care to outpatient or home settings, the types of clinicians and services needed by patients are changing. Only the most acutely ill patients remain in the hospital. This trend raises the demand for increased ambulatory and home care services and providers. In response, health care clinicians need to develop a much more "transparent and boundary-less" system to provide the care that meets patients' needs and preferences regardless of the setting (Wolf & Greenhouse, 2007, p. 383). Seeking out best practices through such EBP strategies as review-ing current research, contacting other health care facilities, analyzing quality improvement data, and garnering patient feedback can support an organiza-tion in developing processes for ensuring that patients are better prepared for discharge, that effective systems are in place to facilitate home health care ser-vices, and that mechanisms are in place to ensure a seamless hand-off between inpatient and outpatient providers.

Advances in Medicine

The rapid and continuous growth in new technology requires health care clini-cians to spend more time updating their knowledge, expertise, and skills to provide the most effective care for patients. Using an EBP approach can help narrow down key clinical questions related to new technology and can assist a health care organization in identifying if a specific technology is a good fit for the organization and the intended patient population. EBP can also be effective in identifying new teaching strategies, such as the use of simulation centers, online interactive educational programs, or webinars.

Advances in IT

Major changes in practice, which affect all disciplines, have been brought about by increased computerization—for example, new clinical information inter-faces, improved methods of data analysis, telehealth, and remote monitoring of patients. Implementing new IT programs can present major challenges to organizations. One example is the conversion from paper to online: paperless medical record systems. EBP can help identify how other organizations have implemented such a significant change, the costs involved, the best educational approaches, and even staffing requirements. An EBP approach can also help identify the effectiveness of new approaches, such as remote monitoring of acute care patients from an ICU within a particular hospital or remote monitoring of patients between hospitals across town or around the world.

Changes in Reimbursement

Hospitals are being faced with a decline in traditional reimbursement and a move toward reimbursement tied to performance. Organizations are challenged to reduce inefficiency and to focus on evidence-based strategies that can improve patient care outcomes. This serious focus on reducing health care waste, improving patient satisfaction, and enhancing patient safety is predicted to continue far into the future.

EBP and the Magnet Journey: A New Vision

Magnet designation is a significant impetus in the development of EBP cultures in many health care organizations. "Magnet organizations have an ethical and professional responsibility to contribute to patient care, the organization, and the profession in terms of new knowledge, innovation, and improvements" (Wolf, Triolo, & Ponte, 2008, p. 203). Current systems need to be constantly evolving to be successful in the future.

The new Magnet model (ANCC, 2008) reconfigures the original 14 Forces of Magnetism into 5 model components:

1. Transformational leadership

2. Structural empowerment

3. Exemplary professional practice

4. New knowledge, innovation, and improvements

5. Empirical quality results

The new vision was created to underscore "the importance of Magnet organizations in shaping future changes essential to the continued development of the nursing profession and to quality outcomes in patient care" (ANCC, 2008, p. 3). Magnet-recognized organizations serve as a major source of knowledge and expertise for the delivery of nursing care around the world and are characterized by their focus on discovery and innovation. An EBP approach is intertwined throughout the five components of the Magnet model.

Transformational Leadership

In the first component, transformational leadership, nurse leaders are charged with transforming organizations to be in the best possible position for the future. "The intent is no longer to just solve problems, fix broken systems, and empower staff, but to actually transform the organization to meet the future" (Wolf, Triolo, & Ponte, 2008, p. 202). This requires creating an environment that is innovative, fosters continuous inquiry, and supports knowledge development and translation within the work setting. This knowledge informs efforts to continuously improve both clinical and organizational processes and outcomes (RNAO, 2006). Therefore, transformational nurse leaders must model the use of evidence-based decision making in their everyday practice. These leaders must ensure that staff members have the resources (human, technical, financial) to support the development of EBP knowledge and skills, carry out EBP projects, and disseminate EBP findings both internally and externally.

Structural Empowerment

Structural empowerment, the second model component, includes the promotion of an "innovative environment where strong professional practice flourishes and where the mission, vision, and values come to life to achieve the outcomes believed to be important for the organization. Staff members need to be developed, directed, and empowered to find the best way to accomplish the organizational goals and desired outcomes" (ANCC, 2008, p. 5). EBP encourages staff to continually question nursing and organizational practice and to ask whether or not they are achieving the best possible outcomes for both their patients and the organization. It provides a structured process for seeking out best practices across the globe. Through the use of EBP, staff members become empowered to change practice based on scientific evidence, thereby promoting increased autonomy and professionalism.

Exemplary Professional Practice

The third model component, exemplary professional practice, embodies the true essence of Magnet. It includes "a comprehensive understanding of the role of nursing, the application of that role with patients, families, communities, the interdisciplinary team, and the application of new knowledge and evidence" (ANCC, 2008, p. 5). EBP integrates knowledge into clinical and operational processes, transforming scientific findings into recommendations for practice and implementing quality processes to change practice and monitor outcomes (Reigle, Stevens, Belcher, Huth, McGuire, et al., 2008). EBP provides the foundation for nursing's role and professional practice.

An EBP approach is also critical in how staff members are educated and prepared to meet future challenges in nursing and health care, encompassing both academic and continuing education within the health care setting. Traditional educational strategies that have been used for decades need to be evaluated in light of "best practices" to better meet the learning needs of multigenerational staff.

New Knowledge, Innovation, and Improvements

New knowledge, innovation, and improvements, the fourth model component, set forth the ethical and professional responsibility of nursing to contribute to patient care, the organization, and the profession in terms of each of these components. This responsibility comprises "new models of care, application of existing evidence and new evidence, and visible contributions to the science of nursing" (ANCC, 2008, p. 6). Research generates new knowledge for the nursing profession. The EBP process can result in several outcomes—it identifies best practices that can serve to prompt a change in practice, evaluates new evidence to validate existing practice, or identifies a gap in knowledge necessitating a need for additional research. Organizations that have incorporated EBP within the work setting often see an increase in nursing research activities as a result of nurses using EBP to highlight gaps in scientific knowledge. In addition, the EBP process promotes internal and external dissemination of findings through various means of communication, such as poster presentations, podium presentations, and journal articles.

Empirical Quality Results

The fifth model component, empirical quality results, describes a shift from what is being done to the outcomes achieved. With the introduction of this component, the Magnet Recognition Program is now placing particular emphasis on the difference that a specific change has made. Outcomes might be related to nursing, the workforce, patients, or the organization. This component involves quantitative measurement, for example, metric selection, data collection, and benchmarking. The EBP process supports the use of various sources of data (for example, quality improvement, financial analysis, and program evaluation) as evidence when the organization is answering an EBP question. In addition, the EBP process recommends the development of outcome measures to monitor and evaluate resultant practice changes.

Case in Point

Roles of Leaders and Front-Line Nurses

The need to develop a culture that supports the use of EBP in today's health care setting is clearly apparent. Transformational leadership is required to establish the vision, provide direction, and empower staff. Transformational leaders "promote employee development, attend to needs and motives of followers, inspire through optimism, influence changes in perception, provide intellectual stimulation, and encourage follower creativity" (Tomey, 2009, p. 187). Nurse leaders must inspire, both in word and action, the incorporation of evidence into practice. Their task is painting the vision that EBP is a process that can be learned and used by every level of nurse within their organizations.

Bedside clinicians, those who experience firsthand the clinical outcomes of their care, especially need to be well versed in identifying pertinent clinical questions for improving care, obtaining and appraising evidence, and determining the appropriateness of translating the evidence into practice. Bedside clinicians have the ability to make a major impact on the quality of nursing care because of the special relationships they build with patients and their families. These front-line nurses are keenly aware of the special needs of patients and families they provide care to on a daily basis. However, they often need leadership, guidance, and an understanding of the EBP process to enable them to identify best practices for improving patient outcomes.

The Johns Hopkins Nursing Evidence-Based Practice Model

The Johns Hopkins Nursing Evidence-Based Practice (JHNEBP) Model was initially designed as a clinical decision-making model for bedside clinical nurses. However, the model has proven to be effective not only for clinical practice questions, but also for administrative, operational, and educational questions. The JHNEBP Model (Figure 1.1) illustrates the concept that a core of evidence, both research and non-research, is at the center of and supports professional nursing (i.e., nursing practice, education, and research). The model depicts the organization as an open system and recognizes the many influences, internal and external, that affect the need for, and the organization's ability to implement, EBP.

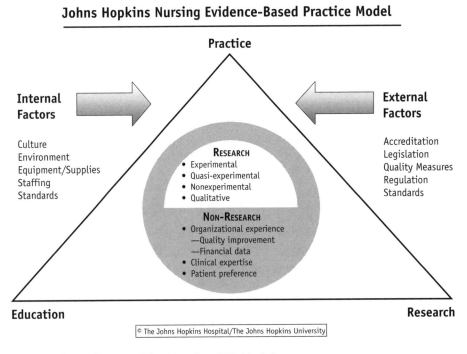

Figure 1.1: The Johns Hopkins Nursing EBP Model

Implementing EBP within an organization requires (1) a culture that believes that EBP leads to optimal patient outcomes, (2) strong leadership support at all levels with the necessary resource allocation (human, technological, and financial) to sustain the process, and (3) the establishment of clear expectations by incorporating EBP in standards and job descriptions (Newhouse, Dearholt, Poe, Pugh, & White, 2007).

The JHNEBP process (Figure 1.2) was designed in three phases to provide the clinician with a step-by-step guide for (1) developing a **P**ractice Question of importance to the clinician; (2) locating and appraising the **E**vidence; and (3) **T**ranslating the evidence into practice. The acronym **PET** provides an easy means for remembering each phase.

The Johns Hopkins Evidence-Based Practice Process
PET (Practice Question-Evidence-Translation)

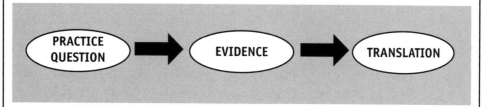

PRACTICE QUESTION

STEP 1:   Identify an EBP question

STEP 2:   Define scope of practice question

STEP 3:   Assign responsibility for leadership

STEP 4:   Recruit multidisciplinary team

STEP 5:   Schedule team conference

EVIDENCE

STEP 6:   Conduct internal and external search for evidence

STEP 7:   Appraise all types of evidence

STEP 8:   Summarize evidence

STEP 9:   Rate strength of evidence

STEP 10: Develop recommendations for change in processes or systems of care based on the strength of evidence

TRANSLATION

STEP 11: Determine appropriateness and feasibility of translating recommendations into the specific practice setting

STEP 12: Create action plan

STEP 13: Implement the change

STEP 14: Evaluate outcomes

STEP 15: Report results of preliminary evaluation to decision makers

STEP 16: Secure support from decision makers to implement recommended change internally

STEP 17: Identify next steps

STEP 18: Communicate findings

Figure 1.2: The PET Process

Several key points are discussed in this section regarding each of the phases in the **PET** process. For a full description of the JHNEBP model, process, and tools, refer to *Johns Hopkins Nursing Evidence-Based Practice Model and Guidelines* (Newhouse et al., 2007).

Practice Question

In phase one of the process, Practice Question, a team of individuals with an interest in a particular practice question work together to define a problem, develop an EBP question related to the problem, and then narrow the question to make it easier to search for evidence. The PICO approach used by Sackett, Straus, Richardson, Rosenberg, and Haynes (2000), authorities in the development of evidence-based medicine, directs the group to narrow down the (1) Patient, population, or problem; (2) Intervention; (3) Comparison with other interventions, if appropriate; and (4) desired Outcomes.

Specific emphasis is placed on forming a multidisciplinary team as early in the process as possible. Having representation from all members of the health care team who are affected by the practice question—the stakeholders—is critically important. Members from other disciplines might assist in clarifying the question and might bring additional insights and perspectives when appraising the evidence. If, as a result of the evidence review, a practice change is warranted, having the affected disciplines involved from the onset helps ensure their understanding and support for the practice change. In addition, EBP group members often champion the need for practice changes among their fellow colleagues, facilitating the change process.

Another key focus point in this phase is the identification of an EBP group leader. At least one member of the group needs to take the lead in setting up initial and ongoing group meetings with team members. The leader divides up the work, monitors the group's progress, and helps keep the project on track. The leader should have a good understanding of the **PET** process and be able to provide support and incidental training as the group proceeds in the examination of the EBP question.

Evidence

In the Evidence phase, the team first identifies where to look for evidence. This step always includes a thorough literature search, as well as a search for other types of evidence (for example, clinical practice guidelines, position statements from professional organizations, quality improvement and risk management data, expert opinion, patient preferences, and community standards). The team then critically appraises all evidence for both its strength and quality (Tables 1.1 and 1.2). They then summarize the individual evidence and determine the overall findings, strength, and quality of the body of evidence.

Table 1.1: JHNEBP Evidence Strength Rating Scale

Johns Hopkins Nursing Evidence-Based Practice

Strength of Evidence Rating Scale

- Level I— Experimental study/RCT or meta-analysis of RCTs

- Level II—Quasi-experimental study

- Level III—Nonexperimental or qualitative study

- Level IV—Opinion of nationally recognized experts based on scientific evidence or consensus panel (includes systematic reviews, clinical practice guidelines)

- Level V—Opinion of expert based on experiential evidence (includes case studies, literature reviews, organizational experience, clinical expertise, quality improvement, financial data, or the opinion of a nationally recognized expert based on personal experience)

© The Johns Hopkins Hospital/The Johns Hopkins University

Table 1.2: JHNEBP Evidence Quality Rating Scale

Johns Hopkins Nursing Evidence-Based Practice Quality of Evidence Rating Scale		
a. High	Scientific	Consistent results with sufficient sample size, adequate control, and definitive conclusions; consistent recommendations based on extensive literature review that includes thoughtful reference to scientific evidence.
	Summative reviews	Well-defined, reproducible search strategies; consistent results with sufficient numbers of well-defined studies; criteria-based evaluation of overall scientific strength and quality of included studies; definitive conclusions.
	Experiential	Expertise is clearly evident.
b. Good	Scientific	Reasonably consistent results, sufficient sample size, some control, with fairly definitive conclusions; reasonably consistent recommendations based on fairly comprehensive literature review that includes some reference to scientific evidence.
	Summative reviews	Reasonably thorough and appropriate search; reasonably consistent results with sufficient numbers of well-defined studies; evaluation of strengths and limitations of included studies; fairly definitive conclusions.
	Experiential	Expertise appears to be credible.
c. Low quality or major flaws	Scientific	Little evidence with inconsistent results, insufficient sample size; conclusions cannot be drawn.
	Summative reviews	Undefined, poorly defined, or limited search strategies; insufficient evidence with inconsistent results; conclusions cannot be drawn.
	Experiential	Expertise is not discernable or is dubious.

Translation

In the last phase, Translation, the EBP team determines if the evidence is strong enough and of sufficient quality to warrant a change in practice. If a practice change is recommended, this change is often implemented by means of a small-scale pilot. Developing and monitoring outcomes during the pilot are critically important. If outcome measures are met, the team continues to work with organizational leaders to implement the change on a larger scale. They then report the results of the EBP project both within the organization and externally.

Internally, other departments might be interested in implementing the practice change within their settings. External reporting on the results of EBP projects at conferences, meetings, or through journal articles helps to educate others about the EBP process and to translate research and evidence into practice on a global scale. Once again, the role of the transformational leader is front and center, ensuring that team members have the financial support, human and material resources, knowledge, and encouragement needed to conduct the EBP project, to translate the findings into practice, and to disseminate the findings both inside and outside the organization.

Case in Point

Transforming Outpatient Nursing Practice Through Evidence

The Johns Hopkins Outpatient Center (JHOPC) is contiguous to a large, urban, northeastern academic medical center and is home to ambulatory surgery, endoscopy, pulmonary testing, radiology, express testing, and 17 adult and pediatric specialty clinics. In addition, Johns Hopkins Medicine treats outpatients in two large suburban centers and several smaller outpatient practices scattered throughout the city and surrounding county. The total number of outpatients treated in these sites annually is well over 500,000.

Over the years, nurses in these settings have raised many practice questions. One question of particular interest to nurse leaders was, "How do we best care for patients coming from home with a history of drug-resistant organisms from an infection-control perspective, and how do we keep other patients from contracting the infection(s)?" Of justifiable concern was the fact that, in the absence of an outpatient isolation policy, a widespread variation in the answer to this important question existed. Nurse leaders saw evident variations in use of personal protective equipment (PPE) in exam rooms; area cleaning following visits from persons with known drug-resistant organisms; handling of patients with no medical history who arrived with symptoms of contagious illnesses; and cleaning of equipment, carpets, and furnishings in clinic and waiting room areas. Nurses concerned with patient and visitor safety and efficient use of resources were frustrated with the lack of clarity about best infection-control practices in this setting.

To address this issue, nurse leaders formed an outpatient infection control committee (OPIC). Membership included clinic nurses, infection control nurses, and physicians from 12 departments and three locations. To better understand current infection control practices and determine disparity among settings, the committee developed and distributed a survey. Questions included the following:

- What type of BP cuffs do you use, and how frequently are they cleaned?

- How often are your exam rooms, tables, medical equipment, door knobs, and bathrooms disinfected, and what disinfectant is used?

- How many hand-sanitizer dispensers are in your clinic, and where are they located?

Results confirmed wide variation in practices—for example, products and procedures used for disinfection, housekeeping norms, and number and placement of hand sanitizers.

Evidence

Sources of evidence included the Centers for Disease Control and Prevention, the OPIC clinic surveys, The World Health Organization (WHO), and database searches (1997-2007) using PubMed, Cummulative Index to Nursing and Allied Health Literature (CINAHL), and The Cochrane Collaboration. A University Healthcare Consortium (UHC) query was sent to learn about best practices of other outpatient facilities affiliated with large academic teaching hospitals. Search terms included the following: outpatient, infection control, ambulatory, environmental cleaning, disinfection, Methicillin-resistant staphylococcus aureus (MRSA), Vancomycin-resistant enterococci (VRE), infectious disease, isolation, and precautions. The committee reviewed 19 articles: three prospective studies, two systematic reviews, two descriptive studies, and 12 expert opinion papers.

Overall quality of research evidence was good, and the committee drew the following conclusions. Challenges specific to outpatient settings are affecting adherence to established infection control procedures. These challenges include variability in staff qualifications, minimal staffing model, large patient volumes with rapid turnover, fewer air turnovers (number of complete air exchanges within a building with outside air) compared to inpatient settings, variability in housekeeping personnel roles in different satellite locations, budget constraints related to decreasing revenue with potential overuse of some supplies, and limited staff education time. Experts identified a need for policies and procedures for cleaning and disinfection of exam rooms, procedure rooms, equipment, waiting rooms, and common areas that delineate frequency of cleaning, responsible personnel, and staff education on infection control procedures, particularly hand hygiene.

Translation

Despite the lack of strong research evidence, consistent recommendations by experts led nurse leaders on the OPIC to draft an outpatient infection control policy that addressed the following:

- Using standard precautions with all patients.

- Having PPE and instructions for use available in all outpatient settings.

- Scheduling patients with known contagious illness as the last appointment of the day and escorting these patients directly to exam rooms.

- Disinfecting all surfaces and patient equipment at least daily, after each patient with possible or known contagious illness, and when visibly soiled.

- Promoting respiratory etiquette and proper hand hygiene.

Nurse leaders were influential in procuring the support of the stakeholders to facilitate passage of the policy through medical board committees. Their persistence and diligence paid off, despite encountering resistance from physicians who had concerns about the ability of current staffing levels to meet cleaning and disinfection requirements, the loss of efficiencies in patient flow, and the practicality of health care workers donning a mask for all patients with respiratory symptoms, particularly during prolonged flu and respiratory syncytial virus seasons. The final policy requires patients with symptoms (rather than health care workers) to wear surgical masks in outpatient settings as tolerated, and to increase supply of reusable equipment in the event that timely disinfection of soiled equipment is not possible.

To ensure adoption of the new policy, nurse leaders:

- Developed a policy addendum that clearly outlines the required frequency of environmental and equipment cleaning and disinfection

- Trained environmental services staff on mode of transmission of contagions, use of PPE, and proper use of hospital-approved germicides

- Provided PPE ordering information to nursing staff

- Procured hand-sanitizer dispensers inside and outside of every exam room, waiting area, lobby, and elevator bay

- Placed signage, PPE, tissues, and sanitizer at entrances and registration areas

- Instituted patient and visitor screening procedures to ask those with cough, sore throat, and other respiratory symptoms to wear a mask

Transformational nurse leadership has empowered staff members at every level to play an active role in preventing the spread of infection in the outpatient setting. Individual staff members now have clarity about how to effectively execute this role. In 2008, nurse leaders published the results of this project in their professional journal, *American Academy of Ambulatory Care Nursing Viewpoint*, and presented a poster at a national conference (Rice & Kubiak, 2008). Outpatient nurses around the country expressed a strong interest in this topic and the guidelines that resulted from this project. When H1N1 surfaced, nurse leaders felt confident that outpatient staff members were well prepared to meet this challenge.

Meeting the EBP Challenge

Implementing EBP within an organization and insuring that clinicians have the appropriate knowledge and skills can be a major challenge. Despite the number of published articles and books on EBP, research shows that many nurses are still uninformed about EBP. A study of 1,097 nurses (Pravikoff, Pierce, & Tanner, 2005) found that (1) almost half the nurses studied did not know what EBP was; (2) more than half reported that they did not believe their colleagues used research in their practice; and (3) only 27 participants had been taught to use an electronic database. A 2006 Sigma Theta Tau International study of 568 nurses found that more than 40% of respondents reported a high level of comfort with the EBP process; 50 percent indicated a moderate level of comfort; and about 10 percent indicated a low level of confidence with EBP. Clearly, a need exists for increased EBP education and the opportunity to participate in EBP projects within health care organizations.

Turkel and colleagues (2005) have developed a progressive model for the integration of EBP as part of the Magnet Recognition process. The model includes (1) establishing a foundation for EBP, which involves the commitment of leadership, incorporating EBP into performance appraisals and clinical ladders, and securing the necessary resources; (2) having staff identify areas of concern (practice questions); (3) creating internal expertise through educational offerings and journal clubs to build necessary skills and confidence to perform EBP; (4) implementing EBP, which involves learning to critique the literature, validate or change practice, and disseminate the findings; and (5) facilitating staff's ability to contribute to a research study.

Facing Barriers to EBP

Although selecting and implementing an EBP process within an organization are fraught with challenges, the actual translation of EBP findings into practice can prove to be even more difficult. Nananda (2005) suggests that two of these challenges are the identification of clinically relevant, scientifically robust findings from published research studies to answer the clinical question and contending with conflicting findings. However, even in the face of robust research findings, additional factors such as the clinician's perception of the benefit of the change (for example, cost, risk, doing the right thing) and its compatibility with existing processes can affect the likelihood of change (Wolff & Desch, 2005). In fact, logistical barriers exist at multiple levels: clinician, organizational, and national or policy level. According to Kalassian and colleagues (2002):

- Clinicians might face time constraints and skill deficits as they attempt to develop a new guideline or assess a body of literature. If guidelines exist, the clinician might lack the confidence to put them into practice or reject the practice change, believing it is not applicable or appropriate to their patients or setting.

■   At the organizational level, the decision to translate evidence into practice might be affected by the institution's willingness to replace long-established practices, even if unproven. Cost is certainly of general concern at all levels, with change being less likely if the practice change is expensive, is difficult to implement, or affects reimbursement.

■   Nationally, implementing EBP change requires tremendous resources, because the change often affects socially and geographically diverse health care populations and environments.

Building Support

The EBP team must gain internal support for the practice change despite the differing goals of administrators and clinicians. Educating and involving three types of people—opinion leaders, change champions, and expert consultants— are critical steps to promoting change (Titler, 2007). Within the hospital setting, research by Bradley and colleagues (2004) at Yale School of Medicine, Epidemiology and Public Health, involving nine hospitals, identified five major challenges that must be addressed to be successful in translating evidence into practice:

■   Gaining internal support for the program or practice change despite differing requirements and goals of administration and clinical staff

■   Ensuring effective clinician leadership

■   Integrating with existing programs or practices

■   Balancing program or practice change costs with hospital-specific circumstances

■   Documenting the outcomes of the program or practice change despite limited resources for data collection and analysis; maintaining the momentum in the face of unrealistic time frames and limited resources

Wensing and colleagues (2006) found that the use of multidisciplinary teams in EBP projects improved patient outcomes, provided improved integrated care services, and decreased costs. Careful assessment of current practice, causes of identified gaps in current and desired practice, behaviors that need to change, and people who should be involved needs to occur early in the change process so that the EBP team can tailor the implementation specifically for the organization (Titler, 2007).

Summary

Developing a strong organizational culture that recognizes the importance of using EBP, educating staff, and providing time and opportunity to participate in EBP/research projects is essential for creating a strong foundation for nursing practice. EBP has been identified as a key to quality and excellence in nursing service. Achieving Magnet designation assumes the existence of EBP and the related research support structures that are a hallmark of excellence in nursing services (Shirey, 2006). Nurse leaders within an organization play a key role in setting the vision and ensuring the necessary resources and support for transforming nursing practice based on evidence.

References

American Nurses Credentialing Center. (2008). *A new model for ANCC's Magnet Recognition Program*. Retrieved October 26, 2009, from http://www.nursecredentialing.org

Bradley, E., Schlesinger, M., Webster, T., Baker, D., & Inouye, S. (2004). Translating research into clinical practice: Making it happen. *Journal of American Geriatrics Society, 52*, pp. 1875-1882.

Institute of Medicine. (2001). Crossing the quality chasm: A new health system for the 21st century. Washington, DC: National Academy of Sciences. Retrieved October 26, 2009, from http://www.iom.edu/?id=12736

Kalassian, K., Dremsizov, T., & Angus, D. (2002). Translating research evidence into clinical practice: New challenges for critical care. *Critical Care, 6*, pp. 11-14.

Nananda, F. (2005). Challenges in translating research into practice. *Journal of Women's Health, 14*(1), pp. 87-95.

Newhouse, R. P., Dearholt, S. L., Poe, S. S., Pugh, L. C., & White, K. M. (2007). *Johns Hopkins Nursing evidence-based practice models and guidelines*. Indianapolis, IN: Sigma Theta Tau International.

Pravikoff, D. S., Pierce, S. T., & Tanner, A. (2005). Evidence-based practice readiness study supported by academy nursing informatics expert panel. *Nursing Outlook, 53*(1), pp. 49-50.

Registered Nurses' Association of Ontario. (2006). Healthy work environments best practice guidelines: Developing and sustaining nursing leadership. Retrieved November 30, 2009, from http://www.rnao.org/Storage/16/1067_BPG_Sustain_Leadership.pdf

Reigle, B. S., Stevens, K. R., Belcher, J. V., Huth, M. M., McGuire, E., Mais, D., & Volz, T. (2008). Evidence-based practice and the road to magnet status. *Journal of Nursing Administration, 38*(2), pp. 87-107.

Rice, M. A., & Kubiak, J. (2008). Evidence-based guidelines for environmental cleaning and disinfection in the outpatient clinical setting. *AAACN Viewpoint, 30*(1), pp. 4-7.

Sackett, D. L., Straus, S. E., Richardson, W. S., Rosenberg, W., & Haynes, R. B. (2000). *Evidence-based medicine: How to practice and teach EBM*. Edinburgh, Scotland: Churchill.

Shirey, M. (2006). Evidence-based practice: How nurse leaders can facilitate innovation. *Nursing Administration Quarterly, 30*(3), pp. 252-265.

Sigma Theta Tau International. (2006). Honor society study shows majority of nurses rely on evidence-based practice. Retrieved October 26, 2009, from http://www.nursingknowledge.org/Portal/main.aspx?pageid=92&channelid=11&HeaderText=Evidence%20Based%20Practice%20Research%20Study&ContentID=78740

Titler, M. (2007). Translating research in practice. *American Journal of Nursing, 107*(6), pp. 26-33.

Tomey, A. M. (2009). *Guide to nursing management and leadership* (8th ed.). St. Louis, MO: Mosby-Elsevier.

Turkel, M. C., Reidinger, G., Ferket, K., & Reno, K. (2005). An essential component of the Magnet journey: Fostering an environment for evidence-based practice and nursing research. *Nursing Administration Quarterly, 29*(3), pp. 254-262.

Wensing, M., Wollersheim, H., & Grol, R. (2006). Organizational interventions to implement improvements in patient care: A structured review of reviews. *Implementation Science, 1*(2). Retrieved October 26, 2009, from http://www.implementationscience.com/content/pdf/1748-5908-1-2.pdf

Wolf, G., & Greenhouse, P. K. (2007). Blueprint for design: Creating models that direct change. *Journal of Nursing Administration, 37*(9), pp. 381-387.

Wolf, G., Triolo, P., & Ponte, P. (2008). Magnet recognition program, the next generation. *Journal of Nursing Administration, 38*(4), pp. 200-204.

Wolff, A. C., & Desch, C. E. (2005). Clinical practice guidelines in oncology: Translating evidence into practice. *Journal of Oncology Practice, 1*(4), pp. 160-161.

Assessing Nursing Leadership Readiness

Evidence-based practice (EBP) holds the promise of improving patient safety and outcomes, advancing nursing practice, and elevating the nurse's role in clinical decision making. However, achieving these outcomes in the settings in which nurses practice requires a transformational change distinguished by effective, involved, and committed leaders.

Assessing nursing leadership readiness for EBP is a necessary first step in implementing this transformational change. Leadership readiness can be viewed through two interdependent lenses: leadership roles and leadership competencies. This chapter provides a road map for assessing nursing leadership readiness by focusing on contextual attributes of the nursing practice environment and the essential leadership competencies to implement EBP.

Context of the Practice Environment

The context of the practice environment matters and can encourage and support, or discourage and impede, the use of evidence in practice. For example, organizations or units might nurture and be receptive to innovations and encourage risk taking, value learning, and create enabling structures, or they might be resistant to change and see those who propose change as a threat to stability. Kitson and colleagues (1998) identify context as a core element in their conceptual framework for enabling EBP. McCormack, Kitson, Harvey, Rycroft-Malone, Tichen, & Seers, (2002) build on this framework through their concept analysis of context which they describe as the forces at play in the physical environment where practice takes place—the interaction of the organizational systems and structures that shape the practice environment. Evidence indicates that complexity, culture, leadership, trust, and staff involvement (McCormack, et al., 2002, Institute of Medicine, 2004) are characteristics of contexts that are receptive to practice change. These contextual factors must be understood and assessed because they are essential precursors to, and enablers for, a transformational change such as EBP (Laschinger, Finegan, & Wilk, 2009; IOM, 2004; Titler, 2008).

Complexity

The increasing complexity of health care micro and macro systems is undeniable. This complexity is reflected in the practice environments of clinicians because of the rapid deployment of new technology, client/patient volume pressures, and consumer demands for quality care and service. Leaders are challenged by this complexity because of the intense demands on systems of care with increasingly scarce resources, as well as requirements for public reporting of clinical, quality, and service performance indicators. These realities exert an impact on the context in that clinicians are expected to provide highly sophisticated care in an environment that is increasingly driven by unpredictability and complex interdependencies among providers and systems. By necessity, the leader's focus has been on reducing cost and increasing efficiency.

Practice based on evidence requires a fundamental change in the way that nursing leaders and staff think about practice and the practice environment. In his classic 1990 book *The Fifth Discipline*, Pete Senge notes that because our mental model has a profound effect on what we see, and because the most crucial mental models in any organization are those shared by key decision makers, leaders must examine their models. Assessing mental models requires leaders to reflect on deeply held beliefs about the organization, nursing and nurses in the organization, interdisciplinary relationships, and how these components interact. It also requires leaders to make sense of the complexity in the turbulent practice environment. Failure to do so limits them to familiar ways of thinking and acting in ways that might no longer be effective in the increasingly dynamic nature of the health care system (Senge, 1990).

Complex Adaptive Systems

The theory of complex adaptive systems (Table 2.1) provides an alternative framework for viewing organizations, for bringing about and planning change, and for understanding staff behaviors and organizational activity. The organization is seen as a complex system "that consists of elements . . . following simple rules, unaware of the complexity they are producing, and making no reference to a centralized blueprint" (Paley, 2007, p. 235). In their influential series of articles on complex adaptive systems (CASs), Plesk & Greenlaugh (2001) characterized CASs as "a collection of individual agents [staff] with freedom to act in ways that are not always totally predictable, and whose actions are interconnected so that one agent's actions changes the context for other agents . . . agents respond to their environment by using internalised rule sets that drive action . . . Rules can be expressed as instincts, constructs, and mental models" (p. 625). Further, "agents change and reorganize to adapt themselves to the problems posed by their surroundings" (Holland, 1992, p.18).

Table 2.1: Properties and Leadership Implications of CASs

Properties	Leadership Implications
Self-organizing behavior of the staff that interacts with, and is influenced by, the environment.	Order emerges without the need for top-down or hierarchical control.
CASs are nonlinear and therefore non-incremental.	Small changes can result in complex or significant outcomes.
Uncertainty and unpredictability of the systems is inevitable.	Create *conditions* in which the desired future can emerge, such as critical reflection, debate, dialogue, and new relationships, all of which might result in new insights.
Complex behavior change emerges from staff following a few, flexible simple rules that are internalized.	A short clear vision rather than prescriptions for action enables practitioners to create their own local solutions to bring about the desired future. Outcomes might be changed either by an adjustment in rules or by the modification of something in the environment, which leads to changes in behavior.

Adapted from Anderson & McDaniel (2000), Paley (2007), Rowe & Hogarth (2005)

Because CASs are "difficult to understand and control—they constitute a moving target" (Holland, 1992, p. 18)—the leader's focus shifts to making sense of the environment, designing a desired future, ensuring structures are changeable, and capitalizing on the dynamic nature of the environment (Anderson & McDaniel, 2000). One aspect of leadership readiness is the leader's capacity to make sense of the complexity in the environment. The organization is seen as an adaptive system that gradually evolves in response to a variety of internal and external stimuli. CASs can help to explain the nature of the change process that is brought about by increasing the potential for natural adaptation and pointing leaders to strategies for sustainability (Rowe & Hogarth, 2005).

Culture

Organizational culture is a major factor in successfully developing or changing practice (McCormack et al., 2002). Schein (2004, p. 17) defines culture as "patterns of shared basic assumptions that were learned by a group as it solved its problems of external adaption and internal integration, that has worked well enough … to be taught to new members as the correct way to perceive, think, feel in relationship to these problems."

Culture exists at the individual, team, or organizational level and creates the context for practice. It is what an organization *is*, a way of thinking about or viewing an organization that is reproduced through social interactions. Readiness for a change to EBP necessitates an explicit process of defining the organizational and unit subcultures in terms of prevailing values, beliefs, and assumptions. Making this process explicit is important because culture operates below the surface. Although invisible, culture is a potent force that guides, constrains, and stabilizes the behavior of group members through shared group norms (Schein, 2004).

Certain cultures are more conducive to practice based on evidence. Austin and Claassen (2008) identified five components of organizational culture supportive of EBP: leadership, staff involvement, teamwork, organizational resources, and readiness to become a learning organization. Large, complex organizations such as those found in health care often have a dominant culture with coexisting subcultures based on professional, departmental, or geographical (caregiving units) lines (Scott, Mannion, Davies, & Marshall, 2003). Though subcultures might share or enhance the core organizational values, they might also adopt incongruent or conflicting values. Scott et al. (2003) identify three types of subcultures: enhancing cultures, orthogonal cultures, and counter cultures (Table 2.2).

Table 2.2: Types of Organizational Subcultures

Subculture	Description
Enhancing culture	Members hold core values, beliefs, and assumptions that are aligned with the dominate organizational culture and they are often more impassioned. Specialty units, for example.
Orthogonal culture	Members accept the organizational values, beliefs, and assumptions as well as espouse their own professional values, beliefs, and assumptions. Department of nursing values, for example.
Counter culture	Members hold values, beliefs, and assumptions that directly question the dominant organizational culture. Groups with competing priorities, for example.

Adapted from Scott, Mannion, Davies, & Marshall, 2003

In any cultural transformation such as EBP, leadership plays a central role in shaping and defining culture by providing a context where ideas, dialogue, and desired behaviors are more highly valued (Scott-Findlay & Golden-Biddle, 2005). When leaders understand culture in the context of practice, it provides direction for how best to bring about change and increases the likelihood that the change is going to be meaningful and lasting (McCormack et al., 2002).

Transformational Leadership

For the past two decades, research has shown that Magnet hospitals have a significant impact on nursing practice and patient care, and now Magnet designation is internationally recognized as the hallmark of excellence for nursing practice and good patient outcomes. Transformational leadership and the integration of evidence into practice, two of the five domains in the Magnet model (Wolf, Triolo, & Ponte, 2008), are critical organizational attributes for the Magnet journey and for managing the unprecedented change occurring in health care.

Emerging evidence indicates that implementing EBP fundamentally challenges and shifts commonly held beliefs about the practice of nursing (Gifford, Davies, Edwards, Griffin, & Lybanon, 2007; Newhouse, Dearholt, Poe, Pugh, & White, 2007; Titler, 2008). Leadership that is intimately tied to this type of fundamental change is characterized as transformational leadership. Transformational leadership is based on a relationship between the leader and followers where leaders engage with followers in pursuit of shared goals (Burns, 1978); are able to see, act on, and satisfy followers' values and motivations in addition to their own (IOM, 2004); and where both leader and follower are inspired by something higher than their own self-interests.

Characteristics of Transformational Leaders

Carless, Wearing, and Mann (2000) researched behaviors of transformational leaders and concluded that the transformational leader communicates a clear and positive vision; develops staff; provides support through encouragement and recognition; empowers staff by fostering trust, involvement, and cooperation among team members; is innovative and encourages thinking in new ways and questioning assumptions; leads by example; and is charismatic and inspires others to be highly competent. Out of this work came the Global Transformational Leadership Scale, which was designed to measure transformational leadership behaviors.

Other valid and reliable tools have been developed to measure competencies associated with transformational leadership. Kouzes and Posner (2003) developed the Leadership Practices Inventory, a 360-degree leadership assessment tool that measures mastery of five practices of exemplary (transformational) leadership: modeling the way, inspiring a shared vision, challenging the process, enabling others to act, and encouraging the heart. Another 360-degree leadership tool, the Multifactor Leadership Questionnaire (MLQ-Form 5X), measures three dimensions of transformational leadership: charismatic behaviors, individual development, and intellectual stimulation (Antonakis, Avolio, & Sivasubramaniam, 2003).

Transformational leadership results in positive organizational outcomes. Cummings and colleagues (2008, 2009) conducted two extensive systematic literature reviews to examine factors that contribute to leadership and relationships between various leadership styles and nursing workforce and health care environment outcomes. They concluded that transformational and relational leadership styles can be learned and that they are particularly effective in increasing nurse satisfaction, recruitment and retention of nurses, and healthy work environments.

Because implementing EBP is a vision-drive change, the decision to begin this journey sits squarely with the chief nurse executive (CNE). It must be undertaken intentionally, with a full commitment and understanding that a shift to a new nursing practice culture takes time—usually 3 to 5 years to embed. After this decision is made, implementation falls to the collective nursing leadership team at all levels in the organization and begins with a comprehensive assessment of their readiness to serve as change leaders.

Trust

Creating and sustaining trust is one of five management practices consistently associated with successful change initiatives and achieving safety practices (IOM, 2004). Trust has been defined as "the willingness to be vulnerable to the intentions of another and is strongest when parties believe each other to be competent and to have one another's interests at heart" (IOM, 2004, p. 115). Staff's trust in the organization and its leaders results in significant organizational outcomes, such as higher productivity (Rousseau, Sitkin, Burt, & Camerer, 1998); commitment and job satisfaction (Laschinger & Finegan, 2005), positive business outcomes (IOM, 2004); and positive work attitudes, citizenship behaviors, and job performance (Dirks & Ferrin, 2002).

The Institute of Medicine's (2004) landmark report on transforming the nurse's work environment provides a review of the evidence to support trust as a critical contextual and transformational leadership behavior. The evidence indicates the importance of trust in organizational relationships:

- Trust links people and groups to organizations, and as a result, staff members are willing to contribute without expectations for something in return.

- Trust increases staff members' capacity for change by reducing the uncertainty and the discomfort that comes with change.

- Trust creates honest and open communication and increases the amount of knowledge that flows among staff.

- Trust can be fostered by an organization's reputation for competence, members' ability to access the expertise of others, and the collective capabilities of members.

- The degree of trust between staff and leadership is dynamic and is enhanced or reinforced by positive interactions over time.

Dimensions of Trust

Trust is an attribute that must be earned through the consistent actions of the leader over time. Trust finds its voice in the interactions between leaders and staff, and at its core, is about relationships built on shared values. In their classic book on trust, Maister, Green, and Galford (2000) offer a framework for trust-building based on four dimensions of trust:

1. Credibility

2. Reliability

3. Intimacy

4. Self-orientation

They suggest that being trustworthy requires that a leader display all four dimensions. Leaders might find this framework useful in assessing their trustworthiness and the level of trust within nursing and the larger organization.

Credibility is one aspect of trust that is most frequently achieved. It is engendered through behaviors rather than through words. Credibility is built on expertise, which includes both accuracy and completeness. Factual information and communication, logic, and others' experiences of the leader are used to assess accuracy. Completeness is perceived on an emotional level and generally conveys a sense of honesty. Among the four components, credibility takes a moderate amount of time to develop.

Reliability is about dependability and consistency in behavior. It is largely about the repeated experience of making promises and following through with actions. Staff unconsciously judge reliability by the leader's follow-through and timeliness on simple actions such as returning phone calls, keeping appointments and meetings, and delivering on commitments on time.

Intimacy is the most effective and the most common source of differentiation in trustworthiness, yet it is also where the most failure in building trust occurs. People trust those who are willing to talk with them about what they feel, see, or think. Intimacy is about achieving emotional honesty, while at the same time maintaining mutual respect and boundaries. Intimacy is more about who we are, and if done well, takes the least amount of time to develop. If done without regard for mutual respect and boundaries, it can have significant inter-personal consequences.

Self-orientation refers to preoccupation with the leader's own agenda at the expense of what is important to the staff. In building trust, the goal is to keep self-orientation low and other-orientation high. Behaviors that build other-orientation include asking staff to share their understanding of an issue, using open-ended questions, focusing on defining the problem rather than the solution, reflective listening, and trusting that as a leader, you can add value during the interaction.

Staff Involvement

Staff involvement in a transformational change such as EBP is an essential component of professional practice and requires a paradigm shift in how leaders, staff, and organizational systems interact (Laschinger et al., 2009). Preconditions for staff involvement in decision making are leadership's collective beliefs and assumptions that staff members want to be involved, that they are competent and capable to participate in decisions that affect their practice, and the recognition that they are the organization's most valuable asset.

Leaders become facilitators of the process of decision making for this practice change. They must "be able to create a safe and developmental context for both the staff and themselves so that trials associated with a considerable change in the traditional locus-of-control can be safely confronted, and professional practice can truly evolve" (Porter-O'Grady, 2004, p. 1). Through this process, leaders must provide staff with information and shared knowledge and entrust staff with authority commensurate with their scope of decision making. As a result, leaders harness the talents and capabilities of staff through trust and their direct involvement in decisions. In addition, staff participation in the transition to practice based on evidence increases their ownership and sense of empowerment and is a key attribute of learning organizations (Senge, 1990).

Moving decision making to the lowest level commensurate with available knowledge unleashes staff commitment by giving them the freedom to act and try out their own ideas while at the same time being responsible for the results.

This approach is especially critical in times of rapid change because it increases staff's flexibility, learning, resiliency, and responsiveness to the changing demands of the practice environment. Rigid hierarchies that thwart learning and diminish the quality of thinking of the staff, both vital features of the practice environment, also limit the potential for EBP to thrive.

Case in Point

Leading the Way to EBP

Leadership roles vary based on the leader's level in the organization. Leadership comprises three essential functions related to EBP:

1. Create a vision and strategic plan for infusing EBP into the fabric of the organization.

2. Build capacity by ensuring that nurses have the knowledge and skills to acquire and judge the strength of evidence and translate into practice.

3. Create and foster sustainability of evidence-enhanced work environments that are aligned with the current and future workforces.

Vision

In creating a vision of an EBP environment, the CNE selects a team of nurse leaders who are going to have roles in the change process. Ideally, all levels of leaders are represented in the group, including nurse leaders from the front line. In this way, the process of creating a vision becomes as important as the vision itself. During this process, the group clarifies and aligns collective goals, values, and ideals and develops ownership for the vision, which subsequently positions them to communicate the vision to the staff.

The vision should reflect an image of the future they seek to create, a mental picture that answers the question, "If we were successful, in the ideal world, what would we see?" Effective leaders change cultures around a clear, specific, and compelling vision that inspires commitment and stretches expectations beyond the followers' comfort zones. Strategic plans are generated from the vision and identify the major milestones that need to be achieved during the transformation to nursing practice based on evidence.

Capacity Building

The leader's role in capacity building is to address key components to create the conditions for change:

- Facilitate selection of an EBP model

- Build the organizational infrastructure

- Remove barriers

- Ensure EBP knowledge and skills of leaders and front-line staff

- Identify, secure, and allocate resources, such as staff time to learn the EBP process and conduct projects, library resources, computers, and partnerships with experts outside of the organization to complement internal expertise

Capacity building is the foundation for implementation planning, which might be done by the visioning team or might be assigned to a separate group of mid-level leaders. Advanced practice nurses such as nurse educators or clinical specialists are ideally suited for this role because of their advanced nursing knowledge and their close proximity to practice at the front line.

Sustainability

The role of sustainability is addressed by building an organizational infrastructure to support and promote an evidence-based work environment. Sustainability requires a culture that values learning, inquiry, risk taking, innovation, trust, and shared decision making, that sets expectations for EBP in standards for practice and care, that builds EBP competencies into orientation, that develops a self-generating mechanism for developing mentors, and that aligns incentives to facilitate the uptake and use of the best evidence. Sustainability is about creating the infrastructure for a learning organization, an organization skilled at tapping staff's commitment and capacity to learn at all levels of the organization. In this way, leaders actively manage the learning process and modify the behavior of the nursing organization to reflect application of the best evidence in the care of patients (IOM, 2004).

Leadership Competencies

A number of professional organizations and health care leadership experts have sought to clarify the essential competencies for successful leadership. The American Organization of Nurse Executives (2005) suggests that these competencies include communication and relationship building, knowledge of the health care environment, leadership, professionalism, and business skills. The Robert Wood Johnson Foundation (Morjikian & Bellack, 2005) identifies the following leadership competencies as crucial for thriving in today's emerging health care system: interpersonal and communication effectiveness, risk taking and creativity, self-knowledge, inspiring and leading change, and strategic vision. Transformational leadership, advocated by the American Nurses' Credentialing Center's Magnet Recognition Program, demands "emotional intelligence, rationality, motivational skills, empathy and inspirational qualities and the intellectual qualities of strategic sensing, analytical skills and self-confidence in public presentation" (McCormack et al., 2002, p. 99).

Carroll (2005) studied skills and attributes identified by nurse executives and female leaders and uncovered six common themes: personal integrity (which rated highest and included ethical standards, self-reliance, courage, and candor), strategic vision/action orientation, team building/communication skills, management and technical competencies, people skills, and personal survival skills/attributes. Begun & White (2008) enriched the leadership literature by identifying competencies for meeting the challenges of health care settings as complex adaptive systems, which include shared sensemaking, exploring, and connecting. Finally, there has been attention to the importance of the ethical competency of stewardship in informing meaningful change in practice (Murphy, 2009).

Leadership nursing competencies for 2020 have also been defined (Huston, 2008). These essential skills are identified as

- Possessing a global perspective on health care and nursing issues.
- Acquiring technology skills that enable mobile and portable relationships.
- Having expert empirically based decision-making skills.
- Being able to create an organizational culture of quality and safety.
- Being politically savvy.

- Demonstrating highly collaborative team-building skills.

- Balancing authenticity and performance expectations.

- Being able to envision possibilities and proactively adapt to change and chaos.

All of the aforementioned competencies are critical to success in all aspects of the leadership role. The following discussion centers around seven key competencies that are particularly important when assessing leadership readiness for EBP:

1. Critical thinking

2. Strategic visioning

3. Inspiring and leading change

4. Relationship building

5. Emotional intelligence

6. Managing complexity

7. Stewardship

Critical Thinking

The nurse leader is responsible for ensuring that organizational policies, protocols, and procedures are evidence-based. Critical thinking skills and the inclination to think analytically are vital to transformational leadership in a complex, technological environment in which nurses must process large volumes of data to inform decision making (Zori & Morrison, 2009). Translation of evidence into practice occurs only after thoughtful deliberation of the fit and applicability of the evidence to the particular practice environment. Incorporation of evidence into organizational standards is the product of judicious reflection.

Critical thinking is a foundational cognitive skill that has a powerful impact on leadership decision making in an EBP profession. Effective leaders model critical thinking through their own actions. They expect and support critical thinking in others. Porter-O'Grady and colleagues (2005, p. 30) propose that the discipline of critical thinking is "simply the leader's systematic and organized thinking and expression in a way that represents disciplined thinking." They describe leaders as creating context grounded in a "spirit of critical thinking" (p. 31) that is the foundation for an open environment characterized by curiosity, inquiry, and exploration.

The ability to critically analyze complex issues encountered in day-to-day operations while maintaining the energy to explore new knowledge, ideas, and innovations is paramount to EBP leadership (AONE, 2005). Facione, Facione, and Sanchez (1994), in their timeless study, found that critical thinking skills include analysis, evaluation, inference, and deductive and inductive reasoning. Nurse leaders process large amounts of information on a daily basis, using these higher level cognitive skills to arrive at decisions and to convey a clear sense of mission, vision, and values to others within and outside of the organization. The skills and dispositions of critical thinking, such as analysis and open-mindedness, are needed "regardless of the nature of the evidence used by nurses, the sources from which such evidence are drawn, and the settings for its application" (Profetto-McGrath, 2005, p. 369).

Table 2.3 outlines critical thinking skills that provide nurse leaders with the tools required to frame thoughts, decisions, and actions as postulated by Porter-O'Grady and colleagues (2005).

Table 2.3: Critical Thinking Skills for Nurse Leaders

Skill	Defining Characteristic	Application to EBP
Interpretation	• Understanding importance, value, and meaning	• Establishes priority for EBP and clarifies impact on people and systems
Analysis	• Identifying structured relationships among frameworks of thought and underlying assumptions	• Examines the basis for EBP questions and translation recommendations • Probes relationships between structure, process, and outcome of EBP
Inference	• Drawing reasonable conclusions from the analysis	• Creates or adopts a framework for EBP through a process of deduction

Skill	Defining Characteristic	Application to EBP
Evaluation	• Appraising the credibility and validity of conclusions	• Builds confidence in translation decisions
Explanation	• Clarifying relationships and underlying premises of conclusions drawn	• Articulates with clarity the basis for evidence-based decisions
Self-regulation	• Refining personal critical-thinking skill	• Develops skill in monitoring and refining personal EBP-modeling behaviors

Adapted from Porter-O'Grady et al., (2005)

Strategic Visioning

The art of envisioning allows nurse leaders to accept the inevitability of change, appreciate new opportunities, develop new strategic direction, and articulate a compelling vision (Ibarra and Obodaru, 2009). Strategic visioning is required for the investment in intellectual capital necessary to the creation of a learning organization or one that is dedicated to continual growth in its ability to create the future (Ceppetelli, 1995). Successful implementation of EBP is facilitated by the leader's ability to create this learning organization where evidence drives clinical practice to ensure the delivery of reliable care (Newhouse & Melnyk, 2009).

An effective leader in EBP demonstrates a personal lifelong commitment to learning through example, considers the impact of EBP translation decisions on the organization as a whole, and serves as a professional role model and coach in evidence-based leadership (AONE, 2005). Senge (1990) introduced the concept of the learning organization and described five disciplines (or competencies) in thinking and interrelating: shared vision, personal mastery, mental models, team learning, and systems thinking. Jeong and colleagues (2006) found a statistically significant positive relationship between nurses' use of these competencies and organizational effectiveness. Table 2.4 outlines these competencies as they apply to EBP leadership.

Table 2.4: Application of Learning Organization Disciplines to EBP

Competency	Defining Characteristics	Application to EBP
Shared vision	• Congruence of organizational vision with personal vision fostering commitment	• Keeps the organization focused on what *could be* in a world of best practice • Extends this vision to others
Personal mastery	• Continually improving personal proficiency to attain goals	• Focuses personal energy on modeling EBP behaviors and developing an EBP culture
Mental models	• Examining deep-seated beliefs that affect perspective and action	• Challenges deeply ingrained assumptions that influence translation decisions
Team learning	• Aligning team members' collective capacity to achieve common goals	• Promotes discussion and dialogue among team members to discover new views
Systems thinking	• Understanding downstream effects of decisions on existing systems and workflow processes	• Articulates a worldview that takes into account the impact of change on the interaction between nurses and the systems in which they work

Adapted from Senge (1990), Ceppetelli (1995) and Jeong et al., (2006)

Inspiring and Leading Change

First and foremost, EBP is about change. It is characterized by a continual search for the best ways to do things to achieve optimal outcomes and translation of these best practices into the health care setting. Leaders are called to serve as change agents whether they are developing an EBP culture, building an infrastructure to support EBP, or guiding adoption when evidence translation results in work-flow redesign. In this era of dramatic changes in health care systems and processes "leadership arises to accomplish three important tasks that are faced by human systems: providing direction, inspiring commitment, and facing adaptive challenges" (Begun & White, 2008, p. 240).

Leading change requires the ability to communicate effectively and with positivity, encourage risk taking and initiative, bring resistance to change out in the open to work toward overcoming it, motivate and retain key people, and create a supportive environment for change (Pritchett & Pound, 2008). Leaders must possess the key attributes of flexibility and adaptability to thrive in changing workplace dynamics.

Effective leaders are adept at motivating commitment in the workforce; creating an environment for change; and creating, communicating, and operationalizing the EBP vision (Burritt, 2008). Empowering the workforce to develop evidence-based ideas and put them into practice is a leadership talent that fosters initiative. Staff members feel that their voices are heard and that their opinions make a difference.

Appreciative Inquiry

Appreciative inquiry is gaining ground as a transformational change process in which innovative change emerges from the social interactions among people within the system (Richer, Ritchie, & Marchionni, 2009). Emphasis is placed on using affirmative questions to create a positive learning environment (Kowalski, 2008). This type of inquiry recognizes that nurses both accumulate and produce knowledge and that this knowledge is a source of innovation and change. EBP extends itself beyond scientific evidence to include knowledge gained through the interplay of the political and social environment, interdisciplinary networking, and collaborative decision making. Appreciative inquiry acknowledges that capitalizing on the knowledge, skill, and experience of the workforce in an affirmative and encouraging manner is one of the best ways to create organizational change.

Relationship Building

Those whose leadership strength is in relationship building have the distinctive ability to create groups and organizations that are much greater than the sum of their parts (Rath & Conchie, 2008). Communication and relationship building comprise a variety of behaviors and skills, including relationship management, behavior influence, embrace of diversity, shared decision making, community involvement, medical staff relationships, and academic relationships (AONE, 2005). To create an environment conducive to EBP, the nurse leader needs to be proficient at building collaborative relationships with nursing staff, peers, other disciplines, community leaders, and faculty. These partnerships are essential for success in creating the supportive infrastructure needed for success.

The ability to influence behaviors by creating and communicating a shared EBP vision is crucial. Leaders who can produce sound, persuasive verbal and written materials to address the value of EBP to patients, clinicians, and the organization are more likely to inspire the changes required for an EBP culture. Nurse executives who are adept at influencing can represent EBP to the governing body and educate board members on how EBP advances quality, safety, and effectiveness of health care. They are skilled in selling EBP both inside and outside the organization.

"A greater possibility for creative and catalytic ideas results from the contributions of many minds working collaboratively toward a common goal and shared concerns" (Shirey, 2007, p. 169). Creating an environment that recognizes and values different perspectives enriches the outcome of EBP projects. The ability to build strong alliances requires a focus on relationship building, communication, and investment in human resources. Inclusive behaviors that engage a diverse group of nurses and interdisciplinary team members to execute EBP projects together result in greater success.

Community involvement enables the nurse leader to develop mutually beneficial relationships with other nurse leaders in the community, regardless of whether the leader is situated in a high-resource or low-resource setting. For example, leaders in small, rural hospitals might not have access to state-of-the-art knowledge resources needed to build and sustain an EBP culture. Relationship building with leaders of resource-rich academic medical centers helps to fill this gap. Such relationships provide a forum for information-sharing, coaching, and connecting that provides benefits well beyond EBP.

Medical staff relationships build credibility and allow for collaboration with physician EBP champions. Much of the work of health care is interdisciplinary. Changes in the practice of one discipline invariably affect the practice of other disciplines. Health care is delivered by teams, so the ability of the nurse leader to engage, educate, and gain buy-in from physician colleagues is critical in maintaining focus on the mutual goal of quality patient and organizational outcomes.

Finally, skill in building strong academic relationships enables nurse leaders in service settings to work in a synergistic manner with nurse leaders in academic settings to ensure that both settings produce nurses who are highly competent in EBP. Without such relationships, nurse leaders of both settings run the risk of either producing nurses with a set of skills that become stagnant in the practice setting or having preceptors who do not possess the skills needed to effectively model EBP behaviors.

Emotional Intelligence

Emotional intelligence, often labeled as common sense, is "the ability to read the political and social environment, and landscape them; to intuitively grasp what others want and need, what their strengths and weaknesses are; to remain unruffled by stress; and to be engaging, the kind of person that others want to be around" (Stein & Book, 2006, p. 14). Viewed as an executive leadership skill, emotional intelligence is a competency that does the following:

- Promotes positive working relationships even in chaotic, dynamic environments

- Instills a passion for excellence and dedication in the workforce

- Inspires trust

- Promotes critical thinking

- Influences people to consider how knowledge is used in practice (Bulmer-Smith, Profetto-McGrath, & Cummings, 2009).

Goleman, Boyatzis, and McKee (2002), in their classic book, identified emotional intelligence leadership competencies in four broad categories: self-awareness, self-management, social awareness, and relationship management. Table 2.5 outlines these competencies, how they are expressed, and their application to EBP leadership.

Table 2.5: Application of Emotional Intelligence Leadership Competencies to EBP

Competency	Expression	Application to EBP
Self-awareness	• Emotional self-awareness • Accurate self-assessment • Self-confidence	• Speaks with conviction about EBP as a guiding value, recognizes own effect on others, and welcomes feedback • Is self-assured, has a sense of presence when envisioning an EBP culture
Self-management	• Self-control • Transparency • Adaptability • Achievement • Initiative • Optimism	• Demonstrates composure in the face of complex change, authentic, flexible in adapting to the challenge of developing an EBP culture, values continual learning, creates opportunities for best practice, and has a positive vision of the future
Social awareness	• Empathy • Organizational awareness • Service	• Is attuned to the emotions that accompany a change to an EBP culture and actively listens to differing perspectives • Is politically astute and uses key relationships to garner support for EBP • Monitors outcomes of EBP to ensure patient and staff satisfaction
Relationship management	• Inspiration • Influence • Developing others • Change catalyst • Conflict management • Teamwork and collaboration	• Moves people along toward a shared EBP vision, engaging stakeholders and cultivating the EBP abilities of staff • Champions EBP, managing conflicts that might arise during the transition • Plays as a member of the team, builds spirit and commitment to EBP in others

Adapted from Goleman, Boyatzis, & McKee (2002)

Managing Complexity

Begun and White (2008) describe three interdependent competencies that enable nurse leaders to meet complex challenges, such as integrating EBP into the fabric of a health care organization: shared sensemaking, exploring, and connecting.

Shared Sensemaking

Shared sensemaking is a term used by Weick (1995) to describe organizational social behaviors that lead to shared situational awareness. "Shared sensemaking allows participants to understand the nature of problems and opportunities and to be able to propose innovative solutions" (Begun & White, 2008). Leaders who are adept at sensemaking learn from past experience, actively focus on events that fit the activities in which they engage, use shared meaning and shared experience to guide organizational decision making, undergo a continual process of refining their understanding, and "when faced with situation uncertainty or information overload … will simplify their information needs in order to make plausible, but timely decisions" (Leedom, 2001, p. 11).

Why is shared sensemaking an important competency for leaders who engage in building EBP cultures? EBP requires teams of individuals who join together to engage in inquiry, analysis, synthesis, and translation of evidence. To accomplish this goal, they need shared understanding and direction. Leaders are called upon to make sense of ambiguity or uncertainty and to contribute to reshaping ever-changing practice environments by enabling continual learning and informed decision making at the point of care.

Exploring

Exploration allows leaders to learn more about the complex challenges they face. This uninhibited search enables the discovery of innovative roles and opportunities that allow for growth and change (Begun & White, 2008). Armed with a global perspective about health care and professional nursing issues, the effective nurse leader is open to and aware of cross-cultural diversity and uses this knowledge to inform choices.

Effective EBP leadership is exemplified in the leader who seeks out information regarding best practices in developing the infrastructure to build and sustain EBP. This trusted leader earns respect by providing others in the organization with the information they need to succeed in establishing an EBP culture. The leader shares this information with individuals and groups most likely to benefit from this knowledge and engages in meaningful dialogue to learn from others.

Connecting

Leaders in a complex environment know how to foster the construction of strong networks between and among the front line, middle, and top of the organization, forging new connections and strengthening existing connections (Ford, 2009). They encourage communication among all constituents and cultivate systems thinking, a shared understanding that interactions among parts of the system generate a cascade of consequences. Nurses, at the hub of the interdisciplinary team, are natural leaders of EBP because they are particularly adept at establishing relationships among team members, patients, families, and the organization (Begun & White, 2008).

Effective EBP leaders help others to see the big picture and to understand the interrelatedness of events and people. They break down barriers that prevent shared knowledge and encourage diverse teams to work together to achieve mutual goals (Rath & Conchie, 2008). They can overcome differences among team members and build rapport. Effective translation requires shared understanding and shared commitment to change. Connections made in the relationship-building processes ensure that the leader moves beyond self-interest, demonstrates respect for the opinions of others, and uncovers the commonalities that exist among diverse factions.

Stewardship

Nurse leaders inform meaningful change in nursing practice and clinical care through their own character traits and ethical principles (Murphy, 2009). The leadership competency of stewardship acknowledges the moral imperatives of nurse leaders. Stewardship is the act of promoting values-based practices that preserve respect for persons' dignity and self-determination and promote equity and fairness (Murphy & Roberts, 2008). Haase-Herrick (2005) presents a practical vision of stewardship as "leaving something as good as, if not better than, it was before you touched it" (p. 115). It involves transforming care by engaging others in determining solutions and actions. In an EBP culture, such stewardship ensures that practice questions are answered based on evidence and that nurses engaging in EBP take into account the context of care and ethical principles when translating EBPs.

To be an effective steward of the health care system and the profession of nursing, the nurse leader attends to self-stewardship through succession planning, continual learning, and balance (Haase-Herrick, 2005). Looking beyond personal tenure, the leader develops a strong group of future nurse leaders who possess the skills and competencies required to sustain an EBP culture. In addition, nurse stewards understand the need to continually develop their own skills and competencies to lead effectively in the twenty-first century, especially with respect to developing practice questions and engaging others in crafting solutions. They do this as strong role models who strike a balance between personal and professional fulfillment.

In discussing nurse leaders as stewards, Murphy (2009) discusses the concept of communities of inquiry, which can be applied to structure learning by enabling nurses to engage in experiences that further knowledge and skill acquisition. This strategy is especially effective for leaders who are developing an EBP culture. Nurse stewards understand that practical application can help to shift nurses' reasoning so that the development of EBP skills and competencies emerge out of real-world situations.

Case in Point

Leadership and Organizational Readiness

In creating the nursing vision and strategic plan for EBP implementation at a 380-bed community hospital, the new chief nursing officer (CNO) and the nurse executive team identified achieving Magnet designation as a key strategy. Magnet recognition was viewed as more than an award; it was a huge change to the organizational culture. A gap analysis revealed a lack of infrastructure for EBP. The leadership team identified the first step to bridging this gap as the development of an infrastructure for EBP. The CNO understood the need to assess both leadership and organizational readiness before embarking on this task. A clear understanding of contextual factors associated with the practice environment was critical.

Nurse Leadership Readiness

The nurse executive team was supportive of the strategic goals and saw EBP as an important opportunity for professional practice development. Nursing directors had long tenures in the organization, with educational backgrounds ranging from diploma through PhD. The CNO identified the need to expand this team by adding a Magnet coordinator and a director of nursing research and professional practice. The CNO was faced with decoding resistance from the nursing directors who felt that the executive team should consist only of leaders with operational responsibilities. The relationship-building and emotional intelligence competencies of the CNO enabled achievement of a mutually satisfactory resolution. The result was creation of a monthly meeting during which the executive team receives input into the EBP strategic plan from the Magnet coordinator and the director of nursing research and professional practice.

The director of nursing research and professional practice role provided a nurse researcher whose skill set balanced an appreciation of operations with research and EBP expertise. This role was instrumental in establishing the framework for EBP; integrating EBP into the fabric of nursing practice; assisting staff to develop, implement, publish, and present nursing EBP externally; and writing grant applications to support EBP and research. Nurse executives restructured the traditional nursing education department, re-classing the Director of Nursing Education position as a Director of Nursing Research and Professional Practice.

Strong leaders were essential to create successful professional practice environments that value and support EBP. Such leaders are tenacious, function as mentors and facilitators, and integrate the vision and strategies of EBP and nursing research into the fabric of the organization. The CNO's leadership assessment yielded concerns about the scopes of responsibility of nurse managers, many of whom managed two units. Some managers had up to 120 staff members reporting directly to them. Despite manager support for the approach for EBP, they would be challenged to meet staff expectations of visibility, accessibility, and mentoring. The CNO garnered support from the nurse executive team for a reduction in each nurse manager's scope of responsibility to a single unit and unit-based placement of nurse educators to support the EBP strategic initiative.

The next step was to assure leader education about EBP, as leaders were approached by newly engaged staff seeking support, counsel, and mentoring in EBP. The Director of Nursing Research and Professional Practice procured a grant to develop an EBP leadership program with six faculty experts from local universities. The hospital matched grant funds to establish a four-part interactive EBP leadership program targeted at nurse executives, managers and assistants, educators, advanced practice nurses, and clinical specialists.

Lessons Learned

This experience yielded eight key lessons:

1. Create the right infrastructure with the right resources to support the vision.

2. Leverage individuals in key positions to inspire leaders to drive the vision and strategy.

3. Assess executive leadership skills and competencies and engage leaders in the vision.

4. Leverage enthusiasm generated by staff and leader education to drive the cultural change.

5. Build on the basics; tailor EBP education programs to meet leaders' expectations.

6. Reward and recognize leaders for their work and engagement.

7. Encourage visible executive leadership participation in EBP education.

8. Report on EBP work to others in the senior leadership team and key players.

Organizational Readiness

In preparation for Magnet recognition, the leadership team established councils for the work of creating and sustaining a professional practice environment through shared governance. Most staff nurses had been prepared at the associate degree level and, as such, had not been exposed to nursing research or EBP in their coursework. The primary strategy to bring EBP to life was to engage and educate staff nurses so that they could share their enthusiasm for EBP with colleagues.

The leadership team also established a Nursing EBP and Research Council to promote optimal patient care and advance nursing science by facilitating a culture of EBP, nursing research, and the integration of evidence into the delivery of nursing care and nursing administration. Facilitating this culture was accomplished by educating nurses in EBP methods and providing support for nurses in implementing evidence-based processes and measuring outcomes.

During the first year, the council was chaired by the Director of Nursing Research and Professional Practice, with a staff nurse as co-chair. The staff nurse co-chair, although lacking in EBP expertise, was enthusiastic about EBP and willing to accept this key role. The council included a nurse educator consultant with recent exposure to research concepts and EBP in her master's degree coursework and volunteer inpatient and outpatient staff nurses with a desire and enthusiasm to learn about nursing research and EBP. The charter of this council included choosing an EBP model and educating the council members about EBP with the goal that these members would function as unit-based experts on how to use evidence to improve practice.

Lessons Learned

This experience yielded ten key lessons:

1.   A hospital-based doctorally prepared nurse researcher is effective in enhancing early adoption of EBP and nursing research as part of the organizational culture.

2.   Council members can perceive the assessment of staff nurse EBP knowledge as threatening. Build on the basics so that everyone is on the same page.

3.   Do not assume that a large percentage of bachelor's- or master's-prepared nurses needed to engage staff in EBP. Assure that leaders have the competencies to drive EBP; create a supportive environment; and provide required resources, time, and recognition.

4.   Ask questions and actively listen to assure staff engagement and understanding.

5.   Choose educators well and assure they have a passion for assuring staff success.

6. Engage staff in decision making related to EBP and research.

7. Leverage early wins and provide staff with the opportunity to showcase their work.

8. Develop EBP internships that provide staff nurses with the resources and time to participate and contribute to the practice of nursing.

9. Partner nursing staff with graduate students to work collaboratively on EBP projects.

10. Build EBP council member roles as supportive of other councils such as clinical practice, nursing quality, and patient safety and other project work that requires evidence-based policies, procedures, and protocols.

Conclusion

Implementing EBP is a strategic imperative for nursing leaders in all settings and requires leadership readiness to create an evidence-based practice environment. This chapter provides a road map for assessing the readiness of leaders to undertake this transformational change by examining contextual factors and leadership competencies vital to embedding EBP into nursing practice and the environment of care.

Understanding and assessing contextual factors and the competencies for those in leadership roles is essential for creating the conditions for and sustaining change to EBP. Contextual factors of importance to creating the learning environment capable of sustaining EBP include building new mental models of health care as a complex adaptive system, understanding organizational culture and subcultures, exploring transformational leadership behaviors, and valuing trust and staff involvement in decision making.

Successful development of an evidence-based practice environment is linked to seven core competencies that leaders need to facilitate implementation of EBP: critical thinking, strategic visioning, inspiring and leading change, relationship building, emotional intelligence, managing complexity, and stewardship. Leaders who invest in self-assessment, individually and as a team, are well-positioned for inspiring and elevating followers in pursuit of practice based on evidence.

References

American Nurses Credentialing Center. (2005). *The magnet recognition program.* Silver Spring, MD: Author.

American Organization of Nurse Executives. (2005). AONE nurse executive competencies. *Nurse Leader, 5*(2), pp. 50-56.

Anderson, R., & McDaniel, R. R. (2000). Managing health care organizations: Where professionalism meets complexity science. *Health Care Management Review, 25*(1), pp. 83–92.

Antonakis, J., Avolio, B. J., & Sivasubramaniam, N. (2003). Context and leadership: An examination of the nine-factor full-range leadership theory using the Multifactor Leadership Questionnaire. *The Leadership Quarterly, 14*(3), pp. 261-295.

Austin, M. J. & Claassen, J. (2008). Implementing evidence-based practice in human service organizations: Preliminary lessons from the front line. *Journal of Evidence-Based Social Work, 5*(1-2), pp. 271-93.

Begun, J. W. & White, K. R. (2008). The challenge of change: Inspiring leadership. In Lindberg, C., Nash, S., & Lindberg, C. (Eds.) *On the Edge: Nursing in the Age of Complexity* (pp. 239-262). Medford, NJ: Plexus Press

Bulmer-Smith, K. , Profetto-McGrath, J, & Cummings, G. G. (2009). Emotional intelligence and nursing: An integrative literature review. *International Journal of Nursing Studies, 46*(12), pp. 1624-1636.

Burns, J. (1978). *Leadership.* New York: Harper and Row.

Burritt, J. E. (2008). Organizational turnaround: The role of the nurse executive. *Journal of Nursing Administration, 35*(11), pp. 482-489.

Carless, S. A., Wearing, A. J., & Mann, L. (2000). A short measure of transformational leadership. *Journal of Business and Psychology, 14*(3), pp. 389-405.

Carroll, T. L. (2005). Leadership skills and attributes of women and nurse executives: Challenges for the 21st century. *Nursing Administration Quarterly, 29*(2), pp. 146-153.

Ceppetelli, E. B. (1995). Building a learning organization beyond the walls. *Journal of Nursing Administration, 25*(10), pp. 56-60.

Cummings, G., Lee, H., MacGregor, T., Davey, M., Wong, C., Paul, L., & Stafford, E. (2008). Factors contributing to nursing leadership: A systematic review. *Journal of Health Services Research and Policy, 13*, pp. 240-248.

Cummings, G. G., MacGregor, T., Davey, M., Lee, H., Wong, C. A., Lo, E., Muise, M., & Stafford, E. (2009). Leadership styles and outcome patterns for the nursing workforce and work environment: A systematic review. *International Journal of Nursing Studies, 47*(3), pp. 363-385.

Dirks, K. T. & Ferrin, D. L. (2002). Trust in leadership: Meta-analytic findings and implications for research and practice. *Journal of Applied Psychology 87*(4), pp. 611–628.

Facione, N., Facione, P., & Sanchez, C. (1994). Critical thinking disposition as a measure of competent clinical judgment: The development of the California Critical Thinking Disposition Inventory. *Journal of Nursing Education, 33*(8), pp. 345-350.

Ford, R. (2009). Complex leadership competency in health care: Towards framing a theory of practice. *Health Services Management Research, 22*, pp. 101-114.

Gifford, W., Davies, B., Edwards, N., Griffin, P., & Lybanon, M. A. (2007). Managerial leadership for nurses' use of research evidence: An integrative review of the literature. *Worldviews on Evidence-Based Nursing, 4*(3), pp. 126-145.

Goleman, D., Boyatzis, R., & McKee, A. (2002). *Primal leadership: Learning to lead with emotional intelligence.* Boston, MA: Harvard Business School Press.

Haase-Herrick, K. S. (2005). The opportunities of stewardship. *Nursing Administration Quarterly, 29*(2), pp. 115-118.

Holland, J. H. (Winter 1992). Complex adaptive systems. *Daedalus, 121*(1), pp. 17-30.

Huston, C. (2008). Preparing nurse leaders for 2020. *Journal of Nursing Management 16*, pp. 905-911.

Ibarra, H., & Obodaru, O. (2009). Women and the vision thing. *Harvard Business Review, 87*(1), pp. 62-70.

Institute of Medicine. (2004). *Keeping patients safe: Transforming the work environment of nurses.* Washington, DC: The National Academy Press.

Jeong, S. H., Lee, T., Kim, I. S., Lee, M. H, & Kim, M. J. (2006). The effect of nurses' use of the principles of learning organization on organizational effectiveness. *Journal of Advanced Nursing, 58*(1), pp. 53-62.

Kitson, A., Harvey, G., & McCormack, B. (1998). Enabling the implementation of evidence based practice: a conceptual framework, *Quality in Health Care, 7,* pp.149-158.

Kouzes, J., & Posner, B. (2003). *Leadership Practices Inventory (LPI),* (3rd Ed). Hoboken, NJ: Jossey-Bass.

Kowalski, K. (2008). Appreciative inquiry. *Journal of Continuing Education in Nursing, 39*(3), p. 104.

Laschinger, H. K., & Finegan, J. (2005). Using empowerment to build trust and respect in the workplace: A strategy for addressing the nursing shortage. *Nursing Economic$, 23*(1), pp. 6-13.

Laschinger, H. K., Finegan, J., & Wilk, P. (2009). Context maters: The impact of unit leadership and empowerment on nurses' organizational commitment. *JONA, 39*(5), pp. 238-235.

Leedom, D. K. (23-25 October 2001). *Final report. Sensemaking symposium.* Command and Control Research Program, Office of the Assistant Secretary of Defense for Command, Control, Communications, and Intelligence. Retrieved November 22, 2009, from http://www.dodccrp.org/files/sensemaking_final_report.pdf

Maister, D. H., Green, C. H., & Galford, R. M. (2000). *The trusted advisor.* New York: Free Press.

McCormack, B., Kitson, A., Harvey, G., Rycroft-Malone, J., Tichen, A., & Seers, K. (2002). Getting evidence into practice: The meaning of "context." *Journal of Advanced Nursing, 38*(1), pp. 94-104.

Morjikian, R. & Bellack, J. (2005). The RWJ Executive Nurse Fellowship Program, Part 1: Leading change. *Journal of Nursing Administration, 35*(10), pp. 431-438.

Murphy, N. (2009). Nurse leaders as stewards: The beginning of change. *Open Nursing Journal, 3*, pp. 39-44

Murphy, N. & Roberts, D. (2008). Nurse leaders as stewards at the point of service. *Nursing Ethics, 15*(2), pp. 243-253.

Newhouse, R. P., Dearholt, S. L., Poe, S. S., Pugh, L. C., & White, K. M. (2007). *Johns Hopkins nursing evidence-based practice: Model and guidelines.* Indianapolis, IN: Sigma Theta Tau.

Newhouse, R. P. & Melnyk, M. (2009). Nursing's role in engineering a learning healthcare system. *Journal of Nursing Administration, 39*(6), pp. 260-262.

Paley, J. (2007). Complex adaptive systems and nursing. *Nursing Inquiry, 14*(3), pp. 233-242.

Plsek, P.E., & Greenlaugh, T. (2001). The challenge of complexity in health care. *British Medical Journal, 323*, pp. 625-628.

Porter-O'Grady, T. (2004). Overview and summary: Share governance: Is it a model for nurses to gain control over their practice? *Online Journal of Issues in Nursing, 9*(1), Overview and Summary. Retrieved February 7, 2010, from www.nursingworld.org/MainMenuCategories/ANAMarketplace/ANAPeriodicals/OJIN/TableofContents/Volume92004/No1Jano4/Overview.aspx

Porter-O'Grady, T., Igelin, G., Alexander, D. Blaylock, J., McComb, D., & Williams, S. (2005). Critical thinking for nursing leadership. *Nurse Leader, 3*(4), pp. 28-31.

Pritchett, P. & Pound, R. (2008). *Business as unusual: The handbook for managing and supervising organizational change.* USA: Pritchett.

Profetto-McGrath, J. (2005). Critical thinking and evidence-based practice. *Journal of Professional Nursing, 21*(6), pp. 364-371.

Rath, T., & Conchie, B. (2008). *Strengths-based leadership: Great leaders, teams, and why people follow.* New York, NY: Gallup Press.

Richer, M. C., Ritchie, J., & Marchionni, C. (2009). "If we can't do more, let's do it differently!": Using appreciative inquiry to promote innovative ideas for better health care work environments. *Journal of Nursing Management, 17*, pp. 947-955.

Rousseau, D. M., Sitkin, S. B., Burt, R. S., & Camerer, C. (1998). Not so different after all: A cross-discipline view of trust. *Academy of Management Review, 23*, pp. 393-404.

Rowe, A. & Hogarth, A. (2005). Use of complex adaptive systems metaphor to achieve professional and organizational change. *Journal of Advanced Nursing, 51*(4), pp. 396-405.

Schein, E. H. (2004). *Organizational culture and leadership,* (3rd Edition). San Francisco, CA: Jossey-Bass.

Scott, T., Mannion, R., Davies, H. T. O., & Marshall, M. N. (2003). Implementing culture change in health care: Theory and practice. *International Journal for Quality in Health Care, 15*(2), pp. 111-118.

Scott-Findlay, S. & Golden-Biddle, K. (2005). Understanding how organizational culture shapes research use. *Journal of Nursing Administration, 35*(7/8), pp. 359-365.

Senge, P. (1990). *The Fifth Discipline*. New York: Doubleday Currency.

Shirey, M. R. (2007). Competencies and tips for effective leadership: From novice to expert. *Journal of Nursing Administration, 37*(4), pp. 167-170.

Stein, S. J. & Book, H. (2006). *The EQ edge: Emotional intelligence and your success.* Mississauga, ON: John Wiley & Sons Canada, Ltd.

Titler, M. G. (2008). The evidence for evidence-based practice implementation. In R. Hughes, R. (Ed.). *Patient safety and quality: An evidence-based handbook for nurses: Vol. 1.* (Prepared with support from the Robert Wood Johnson Foundation.) AHRQ Publication No. 08-0043. Rockville, MD: Agency for Healthcare Research and Quality: April 2008.

Weick, K. E. (1995). *Sensemaking in organizations.* Thousand Oaks, CA: Sage Publications.

Wolf, G., Triolo, P., & Ponte, P. R. (2008). Magnet recognition program: The next generation. *JONA, 38*(4), pp. 200-204.

Zori, S., & Morrison, B. (2009). Critical thinking in nurse managers. *Nursing Economic$, 27*(2), pp. 75-79, 98.

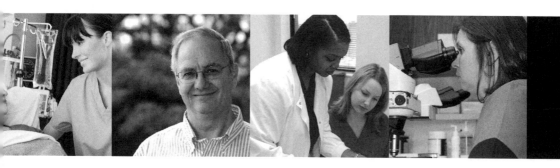

Establishing Organizational Infrastructure

Organizational infrastructure is the foundation on which evidence-based practice (EBP) is built (Foxcroft & Cole, 2003; Newhouse, 2007b; Stetler, 2003; Titler & Everett, 2006). Evidence driven practice is no longer optional; it is a requirement and infrastructure is the essential link that supports translation of evidence to practice (Porter-O'Grady & Malloch, 2008). Without infrastructure, no EBP program can succeed.

Infrastructure is threaded throughout successful implementation of an EBP program, and includes human and material resources that are antecedents to prepare for organizational change (Greenhalgh, Robert, Bate, Macfarlane, & Kyriakidou, 2005; Newhouse, 2007b).This chapter presents strategies to establish organizational infrastructure essential to promote nursing EBP programs.

Strategic Plan Overview

The development of organizational infrastructure for EBP must be approached strategically. The map to building EBP is the strategic plan. The strategic plan comprises goals, objectives, and activities with accompanying budgets to support the human and material resources required. The goals and objectives should match the mission and vision of the organization. The specific objectives and activities guide the who, what, when, and how to achieve the intended goals in a clearly articulated plan. The plan includes realistic timelines, allocation of resources with identified responsibilities, and expected outcomes. Each step includes measurable outcomes so that the team can evaluate the progress and success of the plan. The conceptual (what does it mean?) and operational definitions (how is it measured?) should be included for all outcomes of interest. The first step in the strategic plan is to conduct an organizational assessment.

In Year 1, objectives are likely to include an organizational assessment and gap analysis, budget development, and review of potential EBP models. In Year 2, goals might include mentor education and training and endorsement of responsibilities for groups or individuals. Year 3 might include expansion of the program throughout the organization, incorporation of EBP into job descriptions, EBP training for all nurses, and incorporation of EBP training into new-nurse orientation. Table 3.1 includes an example of activities, objectives, and a timeline to develop infrastructure for EBP. Most organizations have an accepted template for a strategic plan. If you do not have a standard strategic plan template, many are available on the Internet. Use the search term "strategic plan template."

Table 3.1: Example of Strategic Plan for EBP Infrastructure, Activities, Objectives, and 3-Year Timeline

Activity	Objective	Year 1	Year 2	Year 3
Organizational assessment	Assess organizational needs to build EBP program.	X		
Budget	Establish budget for EBP implementation.	X	X	X
Mentors	Develop EBP mentors though two workshops and mentor pairs.		X	
EBP model	Select an EBP model.	X		
EBP process	Define the organizational process for EBP projects.		X	

Activity	Objective	Year 1	Year 2	Year 3
Formalize responsibility for EBP in organizational governance	Integrate responsibility for EBP into committee structure and functions (for example, EBP Steering, Standards of Care, Nursing Care Quality Improvement, Research, Staff Education, Leadership/ Management).	X		
Job descriptions	Review and revise all job descriptions, incorporating responsibility for EBP.	X		
	Integrate changes into career ladder/professional practice model.			
	Obtain approval from human resources.			
	Communicate change to nursing staff.			
	Implement new job descriptions in evaluation.			
Staff training	Provide four workshops for staff nurses to learn EBP process.	X		
Orientation	Incorporate EBP training into new-nurse orientation.			X
Policies and procedures	Establish standard for evidence basis, rating, and grading of evidence for approved policies and procedures.	X		

Effective strategies for building EBP include attention to leadership, capacity building, and infrastructure (Stetler, 2003) and theory-driven approaches (Newhouse, 2007b). Successful programs have been developed (Newhouse, Dearholt, Poe, Pugh, & White, 2007) and sustained (Titler & Everett, 2006) based on careful planning in academic medical centers (Newhouse, 2007b; Newhouse & Johnson, 2009; Titler & Everett, 2006), rural, and community hospitals (Burns, Dudjak, & Greenhouse, 2009).

Transforming Organizational Culture

As the strategic plan is developed and implemented, leaders begin to focus on embedding EBP into the nature of the organization, transforming the organizational culture. One of the first steps is to begin to influence the organizational culture to signal an impending organizational transformation. Organizational culture comprises group-learned assumptions as the organization integrates and adapts to external forces that become an attribute of the group and are then taught as the right way to "perceive, think, and feel in relation to problems" (Schein, 2004).

In terms of EBP, the organization needs to move beyond using single sources of research evidence and organizational experience to inform policy and procedures changes and toward setting the expectation that nursing decisions throughout the organization are going to be evidence-based. Changing the culture and expectations is not easily accomplished, because it requires that the old values and beliefs are challenged. Nurses in clinical and administrative positions alike have to think differently, challenge tradition, demand evidence as a rationale for decisions, refine old patterns of behavior, and acquire new skills in evidence review, summarizing evidence and creating evidence-based recommendations and implementation plans.

Spirit of Inquiry

In preparation, leaders need to prepare for a new way of doing business. This new way becomes reflected in the language used in the organization. The nurses are encouraged to question practice, to ask "what evidence do we have" for this decision and to use words common to EBP work such as *evidence search*, *critique*, *appraisal*, *dissemination*, and *translation*. Nurses are then expected to seek, summarize, and recommend changes based on the best available evidence. For example, practice committees might require evidence summaries with an evaluation of the overall evidence using a standardized rating system. Leaders might require an executive summary that incorporates research, nonresearch, organizational evidence, and patient preferences to support proposed process changes within the organizational system, such as a new preoperative testing process for outpatients.

The spirit of inquiry should be fostered. For example, leaders can set the expectation that nurses challenge any process with no added patient value through formal or informal processes. A formal process might involve new standards review for all nursing procedures. The standard review process may begin to include the rating of evidence on which each procedure or guideline is based. Informally, leaders can model behaviors, such as asking for the evidence that supports clinical or economic value when new products are requested. Leaders have much work to do to enable nursing inquiry and foster a shared vision (Estrada, 2009). A shared vision drives groups to seek and be accountable for a common goal. Nurse leaders can affect both the spirit of inquiry and a shared vision through infrastructure development (Estrada, 2009). Nurses should be encouraged to seek answers to important questions, to work in interdisciplinary teams to summarize evidence, and to make practice recommendations.

A sign of the new culture is the alignment of the EBP program with the nursing mission. A mission to "ensure the delivery of optimal patient care and excellent patient care services" (Johns Hopkins, 2009) can embed EBP structure and processes to support nursing decision making. The nursing department philosophy, goals, and objectives can begin to integrate the new way of approaching nursing and patient problems.

Magnet Recognition

Magnet recognition has been a major force in revitalizing the use of science to inform nursing practice. Magnet organizations are those that are known for excellence in nursing practice (ANCC, 2009a). Evidence-based practice is incorporated throughout the components of the Magnet model: Transformational Leadership (system vision leading to strong professional nursing practice), Structural Empowerment (structures and processes in place to promote professional practice), Exemplary Professional Practice (application of new knowledge and evidence); New Knowledge, Innovation, and Improvements (application of existing evidence, new evidence, and innovations for improvement); and Empirical Quality Outcomes (impact of application of evidence on nurses and patients) (ANCC, 2009b).

Often, the goal to develop a culture of EBP is incorporated into the Magnet journey of aspiring organizations, based on indentified needs from the gap analysis. Development of the EBP program requires a 3- to 5-year strategic plan to create the infrastructure and capacity for EBP if no EBP process or model is in place. An organizational assessment needs to be conducted, and goals and objectives established. Efforts undertaken to build an EBP program are also likely to strengthen the organization's capacity to undertake nursing research, another Magnet expectation.

Organizational Assessment, Goals, and Objectives

The first step in the strategic plan is to conduct an organizational assessment, or gap analysis. Figure 3.1 includes an example of a self-assessment to begin the process. Each question includes an assessment of infrastructure necessary to support the development of EBP. For example, the tool includes questions about whether the organization has literature search capability, available mentors, or access to peer reviewed journals. To complete the organizational assessment, invite nurses from the EBP planning committee or governance committees to review each item, indicating if they think it is present in the organization. The group should discuss the responses indicating the areas of weakness.

Use the organizational assessment to tailor the strategic plan to the organization's goals and objectives for the next 3 to 5 years of the strategic initiative. Table 3.2 includes examples of potential goals, objectives, responsibility, and evaluation for a 3-year plan. Consider the scope of the EBP program within the organization or system. Will the expectations for facilitation of EBP projects be the responsibility of governance committees, units, advanced practice nurses, or champions? Each approach has been used successfully, and the right structure depends on the match with the organizational and program goals. For example, organizations with shared governance councils might want to incorporate EBP facilitation into the council that is accountable for clinical practice. Or, if an organization has an active research committee, nurse leaders might want to begin EBP by placing the responsibility for facilitation with these nurses who are more likely to have some experience with reading and evaluating research articles. If a strong clinical nurse specialist group exists, the organization might want to incorporate EBP facilitation into the group's goals, capitalizing on the advanced clinical expertise and additional training on research methods that these nurses received as part of their master's program education. No right or wrong place to start exists; the important thing is to assign accountability to a group that can carry the mission forward.

Which of the following evidence-based practice (EBP) activities are present in your organization?

	Yes	No
1. Nurses use research evidence to make patient care decisions.	❏	❏
2. Nurses are expected to use research to make patient care decisions.	❏	❏
3. Nurses' job descriptions include the expectation to use research findings in practice.	❏	❏
4. Nursing EBP skills, knowledge and abilities are defined.	❏	❏
5. There is a mechanism for staff to be informed about EBP projects.	❏	❏
6. A newsletter includes EBP relevant topics.	❏	❏
7. Research articles are posted in units that apply to patient care.	❏	❏
8. The organizational intranet Web page highlights EBP.	❏	❏
9. Literature search capability is available for nurses.	❏	❏
10. Article retrieval is available for nurses in the work setting.	❏	❏
11. Article retrieval is available for nurses electronically from home.	❏	❏
12. Nurses conduct literature searches.	❏	❏
13. Nurses use evidence to developing protocols, policies, and procedures.	❏	❏
14. Nurses can critique/evaluate research.	❏	❏
15. A rating and grading system is used to review evidence	❏	❏
16. EBP mentors are available through affiliation with university mentors	❏	❏
17. An EBP consultant is available.	❏	❏
18. The organization has EBP linkages with professional organizations.	❏	❏
19. There are EBP experts in the organization.	❏	❏
20. Advanced practice nurses actively participate in EBP.	❏	❏
21. An EBP or research committee is responsible for EBP.	❏	❏
22. There are unit based EBP committees.	❏	❏
23. Nurses frequently attend research or EBP conferences.	❏	❏
24. An EBP model and tools are in place for nurses to access.	❏	❏
25. Leaders have defined the scope of the EBP program.	❏	❏
26. Leaders are committed to an EBP program.	❏	❏
27. A mechanism is established for nurses to have time to conduct EBP projects.	❏	❏

Overall, EBP is an important component of professional nursing practice in this facility.

Strongly Agree	Moderately Agree	Slightly Agree	Slightly Disagree	Moderately Disagree	Strongly Disagree
❏	❏	❏	❏	❏	❏

What is the educational preparation of the RN work force?

AA_____% BSN_____% Masters_____% Doctorate _____%

What are your organization's goals with relation to evidence-based practice?

Short term goal:_____

Long term goal: _____

November, 28 2009

Figure 3.1: Organizational Self-Assessment for EBP Infrastructure

Table 3.2: Example of Goals, Objectives, Responsibility, and Evaluation for 3-Year Plan

Objective: What will be accomplished?	Responsibility (Target date): Who will be responsible (When will the work be complete)?	Evaluation: How will outcome be evaluated?
Example of Year 1 Goal: Select EBP model		
Review potential EBP models using model critique tool, recommending two for pilot.	R. Smith with subgroup consisting of two people from each of the following committees: practice, education, quality improvement, and research (June 2010)	Model evaluation complete and report to the Coordinating Council in June 2010.
Example of Year 2 Goal: Develop EBP mentors		
Conduct a 2-day train-the-trainer seminar to prepare 10 EBP mentors to lead EBP projects.	N. Jones (December 2011)	Expert in EBP will evaluate skills and knowledge of participants. Participants will self-assess their EBP competencies and learning needs.
Example of Year 3 Goal: Each department will complete one EBP project		
Each department will generate a significant question; search and retrieve evidence related the question; evaluate, rate, and grade the evidence; summarize the evidence; make a practice recommendation; construct a plan to implement the recommendation; and implement and evaluate the change.	Department EBP representative	Each department will report outcomes to the Practice Committee and provide an executive summary.

For example, the first-year goal might be to select an EBP model. The first-year objective would, therefore, be to review, critique, and evaluate potential EBP models and tools to support the process. The objective should include who is responsible for this activity and the time frame.

Case in Point

Finding the Right EBP Model

Recently, an academic acute care hospital conducted an organizational assessment to determine its readiness for EBP and reviewed multiple EBP models for potential use to guide their EBP initiatives (Newhouse & Johnson, 2009). They constructed questions focused on barriers to implementation of EBP, current processes, preferred EBP processes, and alignment of organizational goals and objectives with EBP (Newhouse & Johnson, 2009). The nursing research council set criteria for model selection. The EBP model should do the following:

- Support the whole process of EBP (generating questions, finding the evidence, summarizing the evidence, making a practice recommendation, and evaluating the implementation of the change)

- Include tools to support each step of the process (for example, critique, rating scale, summary tool)

- Provide implementation direction and structure

- Be implementable in the intended setting (Newhouse & Johnson, 2009)

The hospital selected two EBP models and conducted a pilot to determine which model best fit the organization's need. Different groups of staff nurses used the models to conduct a project, evaluating the model utility within their setting. The evaluation tool included direction clarity, tool utility, and usefulness in each stage of EBP (for example, practice question, searching, rating and grading evidence); complexity of the model; capability with the current processes; and the respondents level of EBP competencies and engagement (Newhouse & Johnson, 2009). One model was selected after the groups presented their evaluations back to the research council.

As in this case example, the organization should set criteria to be used for model selection, as each organization's needs might differ. An evaluation tool should be used to provide both quantitative (numeric) and qualitative (words that reflect experience) evaluation to inform model selection.

Major roles for nurse leaders include strategic planning, analyzing nursing issues, providing visionary thinking, and creating environments that produce intended results (AONE, 2005). Based on the organizational assessment, an organization can identify barriers facing nurses in the implementation of EBP, and create strategies to address or overcome the barriers. They can then develop a plan to implement resources based on the gaps identified in the assessment.

Resources

Depending on the structure and responsibility, programs need to project resources. These resources include budgeting for nursing time associated with developing the EBP process, education for staff nurses and facilitators/mentors, and conducting EBP projects. Nursing time associated with EBP activities is usually considered to be indirect time (not direct patient care), so careful planning at the beginning stage is imperative. Programs that do not plan for nursing time to conduct EBP projects will *not* be successful. The positive momentum and commitment to infusing EBP by nurses will be halted and diffused by the inability to participate because of patient care demands.

Mentors

Program leaders must also consider planning for mentors to help train nurses to lead EBP initiatives. Successful EBP programs provide experts to support nurses through the process. Experts in EBP can be trained locally through workshops, seminars, and mentorship (Dearholt, White, Newhouse, Pugh, & Poe, 2008; Newhouse, 2007a) or linked through clinical and academic partnerships (Newhouse, 2007a; Newhouse & Melnyk, 2009). No single approach to develop local experts exists. The important thing is to provide training and mentorship that is appropriate for the development of the local experts within each organization. Some learn best in structured educational programs, so a 1- or 2-day course with follow-up mentorship might be an option. Others might want to be mentored as they facilitate the EBP project or need targeted mentorship in one of the phases of EBP, such as evidence searching or rating and grading evidence.

Seeking external experts to supplement or complement internal resources can be arranged through consultation, part-time or full-time employment based on the organization's need. For example, if the organization does not have a nurse with a doctoral degree or research experience, developing a partnership with a local school of nursing to provide a faculty member 1 or 2 days per week who can mentor staff is a mutually beneficial approach to begin developing capacity and the necessary research competencies.

Materials

Programs also need material resources, including space to conduct EBP projects, tools, computers, Internet access, and library resources. After assessing the resources in place, incorporate the purchase of required materials in the strategic plan so that the budget can be allocated to secure the needed equipment. If not already in place, many of these purchases will be considered capital equipment, with the expectation for accompanying business plans, budgets, and timelines for purchase.

Programs need library resources for assistance with evidence searches and retrieval of evidence. These resources include access to peer-reviewed journals, databases to search for evidence, and library experts who can act as a resource for staff. Often, staff have excellent library resources available, but are either unaware or do not have the skills and knowledge to take advantage of the resources. In addition, library experts might not be aware of the level of nursing engagement in EBP. Forging linkages between nursing and library experts early in the process of building EBP infrastructure has a high return in terms of accelerating the process. In a recent example, nursing and library services collaborated to develop and implement Web-based resources to provide research reports, literature, and other sources of evidence to nurses in the clinical setting (Pochciol & Warren, 2009). As EBP engagement advances, clinical information systems that use evidence-based decision support tools continue to develop (Bakken, et al., 2008). As EBP continues to become part of the standard of care, demand for point-of-care evidence is going to drive organizational decisions for purchase of integrated medical records and systems that are populated with the most recent evidence.

Measuring Success

Measuring processes and outcomes are not new concepts to nurses, who have been central to quality improvement efforts. Attention to defining measures of success during the strategic plan is required for both formative and summative evaluation. Formative evaluation provides the opportunity to adjust the plan based on lessons learned as the plan is implemented, refining and adopting changes based on the nature and needs of the organization and situation. Summative evaluation should be conducted at the defined end point so that an overall assessment can inform the next year's activities.

Metrics depend on the stage of development of the program and objectives. The metrics might include dichotomous outcomes (did we select an EBP model? yes or no) or continuous outcomes (level of EBP readiness based on a total survey score).

Collaboration and Communication

If infrastructure provides the foundation, collaboration and communication are the glue that holds the structure together. Establishing a clear process for decisions and engaging all people affected by the process is paramount for success. Define the responsibility for the groups or persons and map out how communication and feedback are going to occur. In most circumstances, practice recommendations have effects beyond nursing processes (such as changes in fall assessment and prevention protocols or implementation of a new technology), so other disciplines and stakeholders have to be included. Early communication and collaboration can help to make practice recommendations acceptable to all and adoptable. The EBP process should be mapped through nursing and interdisciplinary forums to include all stakeholders within nursing and between disciplines.

Nurses should be engaged in the strategic plan at all levels. Using the nursing committee structure (for example, practice, education, research, and quality improvement) is an excellent way to garner support and solicit input from multiple stakeholders. This might also involve practice, program-specific, and administrative committees in nursing and other disciplines that might be involved in approving practice recommendations from the EBP process. Although many questions or problems are under the domain of nursing, other questions are broad and require a unified approach with each discipline being actively involved in the solution. More transdisciplinary work in EBP needs to be part of the preferred future (Satterfield et al., 2009).

In addition to communication among those involved in the EBP process, communication must also be active with nurses and other organizational health care staff. Use multiple forms of communication to update and inform the organization on the process and progress. Examples of communication media include the following:

- Intranet and Internet Web pages that provide updated tools, examples, and resources

- Newsletters that highlight current projects and outcomes

- E-mail updates to describe new evidence and the impact on care processes

- Poster sessions to highlight successful projects or lessons learned

Organizational Infrastructure

Creating the plan to build organizational infrastructure requires significant planning, assignment of responsibility, realistic timelines, and evaluation. As the plan is developed, a number of activities must be incorporated to assure that the program is resourced appropriately. These activities include education for nursing staff, incorporation into performance standards, requirements for policies and procedures, and integration into committee structures. Each is briefly discussed here.

Education

Regular basic training for nurses and advanced training for EBP leaders needs to be provided. The objectives, timing, content, and instructional design of each session needs to match the needs of the target group. EBP education can be accomplished in class, Web, and online formats.

Basic training should include an introduction to the organizational EBP model, tools, and resources; job performance expectations; and information about how to access resources and become more involved. Completing of basic training should be an expectation of every nurse and can be accomplished in one year through annual competencies. At the same time that the training for annual competencies is implemented, EBP training can be incorporated into orientation so that new staff can receive training. After basic training is completed by all nurses over the year, EBP basic training can then become standard in new nurse orientation.

Advanced training for EBP leaders must also include knowledge, skills, and attitudes associated with the mission, vision, and strategic plan for EBP; EBP methods (for example, reproducible search, critical appraisal, use of rating and grading systems, and developing and evaluating the implementation of recommendations); mentoring staff and leaders, and facilitating groups.

Performance Standards

Establishing clear performance standards through job descriptions, performance appraisals and career ladders is essential to set the standard and begin to infuse EBP throughout the organization. Job descriptions typically incorporate language associated with the delivery of quality nursing care without being explicit about what exactly is required of each nurse related to EBP. Being clear about the expectations for engagement or leadership in EBP and then tying those expectations to a performance appraisal and professional development plan communicates the importance of science-based practice.

Those organizations that have career or clinical ladders to differentiate novice and expert nurses can use the job description to distinguish levels of EBP practice. Others can use one common job description for nurses and use the clinical ladder to differentiate levels of practice. Either way, organizations can develop performance criteria using the organizational template.

For example, new nurses might be expected to define important clinical problems, state their rationale for a nursing process or decision, and complete the EBP basic competency. An experienced nurse might be expected to participate in an EBP project, generating a question, searching, retrieving, reviewing, and rating the evidence with a team and making practice recommendations. An advanced practice nurse might be expected to be an EBP mentor or facilitate EBP projects. A nurse manager might be expected to foster a unit culture that supports EBP and allocate resources for EBP. During annual performance evaluation, nurses can complete a self-assessment to describe how they met the performance standard and construct a goal in their professional development plan, if indicated, to develop to the next step in the career ladder.

Policies, Procedures, and Guidelines

Each organization has a structure and process for the development and review of policies and procedures. As the organizational infrastructure is developed, the standard for use and documentation of evidence should be incorporated. As new policies, procedures, guidelines, and other organizational standards are developed, the evidence source and rating should be included. As established policies, procedures, and guidelines are reviewed at regular intervals, the evidence sources and rating should be reviewed and added.

These important organizational documents have supportive reference lists. These are not necessarily obtained through the rigorous systematic review and analysis of the evidence that characterizes EBP projects. Generally, it is not feasible to conduct EBP projects to fully support all steps in existing standards documents. However, the evidence base can be built over time. The EBP process can be used selectively during the regular review process for specific areas with clear clinical questions. Each time the policies, procedures, guidelines, and other standards are reviewed, pertinent clinical questions can be asked and answered. In this matter, the evidence base of the particular document is strengthened over time.

Organizational EBP Processes

Organizations need to establish organizational processes with responsibilities for EBP. The processes need to fit the organizational norms and hierarchy and link to other committees or persons involved in endorsement or approval of EBP recommendations. This fit can be accomplished by assigning the task to a specific committee or to an EBP Steering Committee comprising representatives who are charged with the implementation of the EBP program. Organizations need to assign responsibility and be clear on the goals and objectives and expected timeline. The next step is to integrate EBP into all of the committee structures and functions (Table 3.3).

Table 3.3: Sample Committee EBP-Related Functions

Standards of Care Committee: Develop and approve policies, procedures, and guidelines that include an evidence rating on all approved policies.

Quality Improvement Committee: Implement and evaluate EBP project practice recommendations that relate to important clinical problems.

Research Committee: Develop and maintain EBP processes or tools and develop research studies when EBP projects do not result in a clear recommendation for practice.

Staff Education Committee: Provide education on new procedures or practices associated with EBP recommendations.

Leadership or Management Committee: Allocate and assess EBP infrastructure and develop and approve budget for EBP processes including indirect nursing time (not involved in direct care for patients).

The organizational infrastructure should be reassessed at regular intervals, at least annually, with the expectation that it be dynamic to meet the needs of the organization and nurses. For example, the plan in Year 2 might assign responsibility for EBP to the Research Committee, where nurses are more skilled in reading research and might then migrate EBP responsibility to the Practice Committee after skills have matured.

Conclusion

Building capacity for EBP requires careful attention to the development of supporting infrastructure. After assessment of organizational infrastructure is in place, a strategic plan is developed based on gaps, or identified needs. Goals and objectives, aligned with the organizational and nursing mission and vision, target strategies to build infrastructure over a 3- to 5-year time period.

At the basic level, these strategies include both human and material resources, which include securing EBP mentors; building nursing skills, knowledge, and abilities in EBP; procuring tools to help nursing staff conduct the EBP process; and developing material resources such as library linkages that provide support for evidence search and retrieval and a documentation system for the EBP process. As the EBP process matures, websites highlighting EBP projects, presentations, and publications and regular outcome evaluation of projects will be put in place. With appropriate infrastructure, nursing staff will be well supported with the foundation for the engagement in and the implementation of EBP.

References

American Nurses Credentialing Center (ANCC). (2009a). Magnet recognition program overview. Retrieved November 26, 2009, from http://www.nursecredentialing.org/Magnet/ProgramOverview.aspx

American Nurses Credentialing Center (ANCC). (2009b). Announcing a new model for ANCC's magnet recognition program. Retrieved November 30, 2009, from http://www.nursecredentialing.org/Magnet/NewMagnetModel.aspx

American Organization of Nurse Executives (AONE). (2005). AONE nurse executive competencies. *Nurse Leader,* February. Retrieved November 16, 2009, from http://www.aone.org/aone/pdf/February%20Nurse%20Leader--final%20draft--for%20web.pdf

Bakken, S., Currie, L. M., Lee, N. J., Roberts, W. D., Collins, S. A., & Cimino, J. J. (2008). Integrating evidence into clinical information systems for nursing decision support. *International Journal of Medical Informatics, 77*(6), pp. 413–420.

Burns, H. K., Dudjak, L., & Greenhouse, P. K. (2009). Building an evidence-based practice infrastructure and culture: A model for rural and community hospitals. *Journal of Nursing Administration, 39*(7-8), 321-5.

Dearholt, S. L., White, K. M., Newhouse, R., Pugh, L. C., & Poe, S. (2008). Educational strategies to develop evidence-based practice mentors. *Journal for Nurses in Staff Development, 24*(2), 53–9; quiz 60–1.

Estrada, N. (2009). Exploring perceptions of a learning organization by RNs and relationship to EBP beliefs and implementation in the acute care setting. *Worldviews on Evidence-Based Nursing,* 6(4):200-9.

Foxcroft, D. R, & Cole, N. (2003). Organisational infrastructures to promote evidence based nursing practice. *Cochrane Database of Systematic Reviews (Online) (4)*, CD002212.

Greenhalgh, T., Robert, G., Bate, P., Macfarlane, A., & Kyriakidou, O. (2005). *Diffusion of innovations in health service organizations: A systematic literature review.* Massachusetts: Blackwell Publishing Ltd.

The Johns Hopkins University, The Johns Hopkins Hospital, and Johns Hopkins Health System. (2009). Nursing and patient care services, The Johns Hopkins Hospital: Mission. Retrieved November 26, 2009, from http://www.hopkinsmedicine.org/administrative/nursing.html

Newhouse, R. P. (2007a). Collaborative synergy: Practice and academic partnerships in evidence-based practice. *The Journal of Nursing Administration, 37*(3), pp. 105–108.

Newhouse, R. P. (2007b). Creating infrastructure supportive of evidence-based nursing practice: Leadership strategies. *Worldviews on Evidence-Based Nursing, 4*(1), pp. 21–29.

Newhouse, R. P., Dearholt, S., Poe, S., Pugh, L. C., & White, K. M. (2007). Organizational change strategies for evidence-based practice. *The Journal of Nursing Administration, 37*(12), pp. 552–557.

Newhouse, R. P., & Johnson, K. (2009). A case study in evaluating infrastructure for EBP and selecting a model. *The Journal of Nursing Administration, 39*(10), pp. 409–411.

Newhouse, R. P., & Melnyk, M. (2009). Nursing's role in engineering a learning healthcare system. *The Journal of Nursing Administration, 39*(6), pp. 260–262.

Pochciol, J. M., & Warren, J. I. (2009). An information technology infrastructure to enable evidence-based nursing practice. *Nursing Administration Quarterly, 33*(4), pp. 317–324.

Porter-O'Grady, T., & Malloch, K. (2008). Beyond myth and magic: The future of evidence-based leadership. *Nursing Administration Quarterly, 32*(3), pp. 176–187.

Satterfield, J. M., Spring, B., Brownson, R. C., Mullen, E. J., Newhouse, R. P., Walker, B. B. et al. (2009). Toward a transdisciplinary model of evidence-based practice. *The Milbank Quarterly, 87*(2), pp. 368–390.

Schein, E. H. (2004). *Organizational culture and leadership,* (3rd ed). San Francisco: Jossey-Bass.

Stetler, C. B. (2003). Role of the organization in translating research into evidence-based practice. *Outcomes Management, 7*(3), pp. 97–103; quiz pp. 104–5.

Titler, M. G., & Everett, L. Q. (2006). Sustain an infrastructure to support EBP. *Nursing Management, 37*(9), pp. 14, 16.

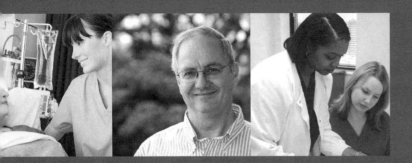

PART II

Building Core Competencies in Nursing Service

Evidence-based practice (EBP) is a core competency for nurses at all levels and in all settings. Nursing knowledge and skills advance continually, and many are concerned that nursing practice is evolving faster than decisions can be made on how to best assure competency in this diverse practice discipline (Ironside, 2008). Despite the challenge, nurses are compelled to contribute in a meaningful way to search for the best practices to maximize patient outcomes. Nurses require specialized knowledge and skills to pose answerable questions, search for and appraise research and other types of evidence, and decide on the advisability of translating evidence into practice. This chapter discusses and defines core EBP competencies for nurses of different experience levels, ties competence in EBP to the new vision for Magnet recognition, describes structures to build core competencies in service settings, and explores ways in which professional development can ensure successful evidence-based practice.

EBP Competence and Magnet

The American Nurses Credentialing Center (ANCC) Magnet Recognition Program showcases a nursing culture of excellence through the achievement of three goals: promoting quality in settings that support professional practice, identifying excellence in nursing services, and disseminating best practices in nursing services (ANCC, 2009). The newly contemporized model comprises five components that both support and are supported by an EBP culture: transformational leadership; structured empowerment; exemplary professional nursing practice; new knowledge, innovations, and improvements; and empirical quality outcomes (Wolf, Triolo, & Ponte, 2008).

Key Curricular Components for Staff Development

Key curricular components of EBP education are linked to the particular model selected by the organization. However, some common elements exist, regardless of the model chosen. Staff development efforts should include communication of the job description expectations for EBP, supportive resources for EBP, and EBP project management, in addition to steps in the EBP process such as formulating a practice question, searching for evidence, appraising evidence, synthesizing evidence, translating evidence, and communicating recommendations. Out of this general curriculum, core competencies can be identified.

Core Competencies for Nurses

A recent systematic review of the concept of competency in nursing found seven defining attributes of competency: application of skills in the particular domain (for the purposes of this chapter, the domain of interest is EBP), instruction that focuses on specific outcomes or competencies, allowance for increasing levels of competency, learner accountability, practice-based learning, self-assessment, and individualized learning (Tilley, 2008). Although the nurse has primary accountability for development of competence in the practice specialty, employers of nurses are responsible for facilitating progress toward ongoing professional competence (Tabari-Khomeiran, Kiger, Parsa-Yekta, & Ahmadi, 2007). Phases of competence development include recognition of driving forces that are either intrinsic (for example, self-fulfillment) or extrinsic (for example, job requirements), provision of appropriate requisites and support for the learner, availability of opportunities for the learner to gain experience in the skill, repeated practice and reflection on challenges confronted during the process, and integration of the competency with prior skills and knowledge so that one can now teach and supervise others with respect to the particular skill (Tabari-Khomeiran et al., 2007).

Cognitive learning can be categorized into six hierarchical steps as first defined in the classic taxonomy developed by Bloom and colleagues (1956):

1. Knowledge

2. Understanding

3. Application

4. Analysis

5. Synthesis

6. Evaluation

Effective planning for EBP competencies seeks to stimulate nurse learners to progressively gain required skills and knowledge as they navigate through all six levels. EBP competence is best obtained through a guided professional development process with a knowledgeable mentor or coach. Guided growth interventions based on Benner's (1984) classic *From Novice to Expert* framework, in which the nurse passes through five stages as he or she acquires clinical experience, have been shown to maximize performance by sharing the expertise of experienced nurses with those having less experience (Nedd, Nash, Galindo-Ciocon, and Belgrave, 2006). The five stages are as follows:

1. Novice

2. Advanced beginner

3. Competent nurse

4. Proficient nurse

5. Expert

Basic EBP Knowledge and Skills

The journey to mastering EBP competencies begins with knowledge. The novice nurse is introduced to the basic terminology and strategies used for EBP within the practice setting and exhibits basic EBP knowledge. Not only does the novice acquire new information, but also he or she can recall that information when needed. EBP competencies for the novice are outlined in Table 4.1.

Table 4.1: EBP Competencies for the Novice Nurse

Knowledge
■ Define EBP
■ Describe its importance to exemplary professional practice
■ Outline the basic components of EBP
■ Identify the organizational EBP model
■ List available EBP resources

After the novice has developed a basic level of understanding, and can interpret most communications related to EBP, the novice progresses to advanced beginner. The nurse now comprehends EBP and can tentatively apply what he or she has learned as an EBP team member (Table 4.2).

Table 4.2: EBP Competencies for the Advanced Beginner

Comprehension
■ Explain steps of EBP
■ Draw links between EBP and quality of care
■ Give examples of evidence-based decisions
■ Describe importance of basing practice changes on evidence
■ Distinguish between EBP and experience-based practice
Application
■ Construct an EBP question
■ Conduct an evidence search
■ Access library resources
■ Recognize basic types of research and levels of evidential strength
■ Use standard tools to analyze evidence
■ Demonstrate effective teamwork skills

Intermediate Level EBP Knowledge and Skills

After exposure to a guided professional development experience in EBP, the advanced beginner is well on the way to developing competence in many aspects of the EBP process. Nurses who are at the competent level of EBP performance can comfortably apply what has been learned into new situations in the work place (Table 4.3). These nurses are more confident in searching for evidence, reading research, using basic appraisal and summarization tools, and recommending changes.

Table 4.3: EBP Competencies for the Competent Nurse

Application
■ Refine the scope of a practice question
■ Perform a comprehensive literature search
■ Appraise research and nonresearch evidence using a standard tool
■ Produce an evidence summary using a standard tool
■ Develop recommendations for changes in systems/processes

As the competent nurse progresses to the proficient level, he or she begins to develop more sophisticated skills necessary for the analysis phase of cognitive development. The proficient nurse can dissect information and examine the relationship of each component to the entirety of evidence reviewed. The proficient nurse progresses to recognizing patterns in the evidence and to assembling the pieces of evidence into a coherent whole with the intent of creating recommendations (Table 4.4). Proficient nurses are active members of the EBP team and are emerging leaders within the team.

Table 4.4: EBP Competencies for the Proficient Nurse

Analysis
- Recognize faulty reasoning
- Compare and contrast evidence
- Differentiate among facts and opinions
- Understand standard types of statistical analysis
- Illustrate gaps in the evidence

Synthesis
- Draw conclusions based on evidence
- Determine feasibility of evidence translation and change
- Create and carry out an action plan
- Recruit and lead an interdisciplinary team
- Construct measurable outcomes

Advanced EBP Knowledge and Skills

Expert nurses possess the ability to put all parts together to form a whole, developing confidence in the cognitive domain of synthesis. These nurses have expertise in categorizing, compiling evidence, and creating processes to improve outcomes (Table 4.5). In addition, expert nurses are independent in the conduct of EBP projects and feel confident making choices based on their review of the evidence.

Master's-prepared specialty nurses, such as clinical nurse specialists, can influence every stage of knowledge transformation because of their multifaceted role that extends beyond patient care to administrative, educational, and consultative functions (Kring, 2008). Developing advanced EBP knowledge and skills in clinical nurse specialists' positions make these advanced practice nurses ideal EBP change agents.

Table4.5: EBP Competencies for the Expert Nurse

Synthesis

- Combine evidence into a cohesive whole
- Reconstruct new ideas based on evidence
- Draw conclusions from sophisticated statistical analyses
- Relate knowledge from one area to several areas
- Organize team activities to achieve goals

Evaluation

- Formulate a stakeholder analysis
- Conduct an organizational assessment
- Produce a project management plan
- Manage a project
- Identify quality sources of data
- Serve as a change agent for EBP

Figure 4.1 presents a visual depiction of the core EBP competencies from novice to expert.

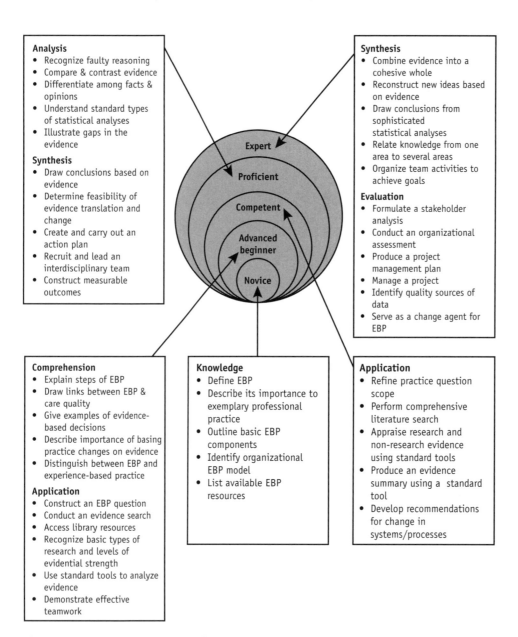

Analysis
- Recognize faulty reasoning
- Compare & contrast evidence
- Differentiate among facts & opinions
- Understand standard types of statistical analyses
- Illustrate gaps in the evidence

Synthesis
- Draw conclusions based on evidence
- Determine feasibility of evidence translation and change
- Create and carry out an action plan
- Recruit and lead an interdisciplinary team
- Construct measurable outcomes

Synthesis
- Combine evidence into a cohesive whole
- Reconstruct new ideas based on evidence
- Draw conclusions from sophisticated statistical analyses
- Relate knowledge from one area to several areas
- Organize team activities to achieve goals

Evaluation
- Formulate a stakeholder analysis
- Conduct an organizational assessment
- Produce a project management plan
- Manage a project
- Identify quality sources of data
- Serve as a change agent for EBP

Expert

Proficient

Competent

Advanced beginner

Novice

Comprehension
- Explain steps of EBP
- Draw links between EBP & care quality
- Give examples of evidence-based decisions
- Describe importance of basing practice changes on evidence
- Distinguish between EBP and experience-based practice

Application
- Construct an EBP question
- Conduct an evidence search
- Access library resources
- Recognize basic types of research and levels of evidential strength
- Use standard tools to analyze evidence
- Demonstrate effective teamwork

Knowledge
- Define EBP
- Describe its importance to exemplary professional practice
- Outline basic EBP components
- Identify organizational EBP model
- List available EBP resources

Application
- Refine practice question scope
- Perform comprehensive literature search
- Appraise research and non-research evidence using standard tools
- Produce an evidence summary using a standard tool
- Develop recommendations for change in systems/processes

Figure 4.1: EBP Competencies from Novice to Expert

Structures for Building Core Competencies in EBP

Structures for building core EBP competencies in nurses include those related to leadership, empowerment, professional practice, new knowledge generation and innovation, and outcomes attainment and sustainability.

Leadership Structures

Translating evidence into practice uproots the status quo and requires leaders who have vision, influence, and expertise in professional nursing practice. Such leaders understand that nursing practice is continually evolving and that learning organizations are constantly changing and transforming to meet the needs of patients, families, and communities. Transformational leaders enlighten the organization with evidence that supports change and generates new knowledge through shared lessons learned as they evaluate the impact of findings translated into practice.

Leadership support of EBP goes beyond financial and human resources for the conduct of EBP. One of eight leadership competencies thought to be an essential part of the 2020 leader's repertoire is expert decision making rooted in empirical science (Huston, 2008). Modeling decision making based on best practices gleaned from the research and experiential learning increases the likelihood of making decisions that result in quality outcomes. Using an EBP approach to management ensures that the nurse leader has access to state-of-the-art strategies to make good decisions and increases the credibility of these decisions in the eyes of professional colleagues.

Leadership development workshops that incorporate an EBP project into learning activities help teach EBP competencies to nurse leaders and serve to enable the leadership group to answer key questions of interest. For example, a workshop might be designed that teaches EBP skills while guiding a group of nurse managers to answer the question of whether or not a link between 12-hour shifts and medication errors exists. Integrating EBP projects into the work of leadership groups, such as management development and professional practice committees, provides nurse leaders the opportunity to practice and hone EBP competencies.

Empowerment Structures

The structural empowerment component of the Magnet model is synergistic to the EBP process. Empowerment, or an individual's positional power, enables successful EBP projects, and successful EBP projects increase empowerment. Formal power resulting from the person's job and informal power arising from the nurse's collegial network facilitate access to four main empowerment structures: opportunity, information, support, and resources (Knol & van Linge, 2009). Evidence-based practice activities provide the nurse with an opportunity to learn and grow, procure knowledge and expertise needed for effective role functioning, benefit from feedback and leadership, and access human and financial resources needed to transform care based on evidence.

Shared Governance

Nursing strategic plans incorporate structures such as shared governance models that empower staff to accomplish organizational goals and achieve quality outcomes. Shared governance is an evidence-based management process model that stresses staff empowerment, accountability, active decision making, and ownership (Church, Baker & Berry, 2008). This model supports nurse autonomy, control of practice and the practice environment, and effective interdisciplinary communication and collaboration. These characteristics are essential to the translation of evidence into practice. Nurses in shared governance environments are empowered through access to information, resources, opportunities to learn and grow, and support for ensuring that their practice is evidence-based (Moore & Hutchison, 2007). Principles of EBP require that nurses have a voice in how they practice, that they not be afraid to question the status quo, and that they have control over their work through critical thinking and autonomous decision making (Zuzelo, McGoldrick, Seminara & Karbach, 2006).

The hallmarks of shared governance (authority, accountability, and responsibility) are naturally compatible with the EBP philosophy. Nurses who work in shared governance environments have experience working in groups and have a skill set that facilitates collaboration and negotiation (Zuzelo, McGoldrick, Seminara & Karbach, 2006). This skill set is helpful for the conduct of unit- or department-based EBP projects. Outcomes of EBP projects within a shared governance philosophy include control over practice, staff satisfaction, and group cohesion, ultimately contributing to decision making at the point-of-care.

EBP teams serve as a bridge between the nurse's clinical autonomy in making these patient-related decisions and the decision-making power of the group, serving as a venue for shared decision making at the unit, departmental, and organizational level (Kramer et al., 2008). Autonomy is facilitated through EBP. Magnet organizations, for example, include support for autonomous practice through active interdisciplinary EBP teams that focus on knowledge and best practices; the products of their work form the basis for autonomous independent and interdependent decisions (Kramer & Schmalenberg, 2008). The Institute of Medicine's groundbreaking book on transforming the work environment of nurses (2004) recommends higher levels of staff nurse autonomy and support for nurses to use outcomes of EBP initiatives in patient care decision making.

Professional Autonomy

Professional autonomy is an outgrowth of the nurse's "ability to critically and analytically look into experiences, to develop and utilize the multiple types of knowledge, and to implement this developed knowledge into practice" (Mantzoukas & Watkinson, 2007, p. 31). EBP encourages the incorporation of both research and experiential knowledge into practice. It is in the translation phase that the EBP team and the individual nurse reflect upon the advisability of transforming the particular evidence-based "best" practice into the care of their specific patient populations or individual patients. Reflection allows the nurse to transform unconscious types of knowledge and practices (primarily gained through the nurse's experience and the needs of the individual patient) into conscious knowledge and practices to justify clinical decisions (Mantzoukas, 2008).

Structures to Support Exemplary Professional Practice

Exemplary professional practice is the application of the best evidence into practice to achieve optimal outcomes. EBP is a model that guides practice, ensuring that nurses exhibit safe and ethical practice as appropriate to the practice setting. Professional practice involves making judgments; making judgments is enabled by critical thinking skills such as questioning, analyzing, synthesizing, and drawing conclusions (Newhouse, Dearholt, Poe, Pugh, & White, 2007). Through EBP, nurses shape and are shaped by the acquisition and translation of professional knowledge. Organizations can use a variety of structures to support this process, including journal clubs and multimodal educational activities.

Journal Clubs

Much has been written about use of journal clubs as a time-proven strategy for effective teaching of reading and critical appraisal of research in clinicians and medical students (Lee, Boldt, Golnik, Arnold, Oetting et al, 2006; Deenadayalan, Grimmer-Somers, Prior, & Kumar, 2008) and, more recently, in practicing nurses and nursing students (Thompson, 2006; Steenbeek, Edgecombe, Durling, LeBlanc, Anderson et al, 2009). An increasing number of professional organizations and clinical institutions use journal clubs as a strategy to foster critical appraisal skills in interpretation of evidence for translation into practice (Thompson, 2006).

With the advent of technology, Internet-based journal clubs have been widely used in medical and nursing schools to provide a flexible approach that is self-paced and convenient (Steenbeek et al., 2009). Although mostly used in academic settings, Internet-based journal clubs would also be an appropriate modality for enhancing EBP journal club activities in the service setting. The flexibility of this electronic medium can be particularly helpful in coordinating system-wide journal clubs, where members are in different physical locations yet are working on a question of interest to all entities in the system. Steenbeek and colleagues (2009) studied the use of a learning management system, Web-CT, to enhance learning through journal club activities across three sites, supplemented by teleconferencing for guided evidence synthesis activities. Articles pertaining to the question of interest were posted on Web-CT and a shared blackboard was used for posting questions. The investigators found that blackboard-enhanced journal club activities helped students who participated improve research-critiquing scores.

Successful journal clubs have a number of attributes that ensure their effectiveness. A recent systematic review by Deenadayalan and colleagues (2008) uncovered the following characteristics: regular meetings; mandatory attendance; clear purpose; appropriate meeting times, locations, and incentives; a trained journal club leader to select evidence and lead discussion; circulation of papers prior to the meeting; use of the Internet for wide dissemination and data storage; use of established evidence appraisal processes; and summarization of findings. These attributes fit nicely within the context of the EBP project, with a trained project leader, a mutually developed project plan, and a well-defined EBP process (such as the PET process).

Another key to success in the use of journal clubs is determining the best approach to fit workflow. For example, organizations have found it challenging to set up and maintain journal clubs in ambulatory settings. Time appears to be a limiting factor, because ambulatory nurses are preoccupied with planning care during clinic hours. Ambulatory nurses have the same EBP development needs as inpatient nurses; hence, organizations have sought alternatives to the traditional journal club format. One research team (Campbell-Fleming, Catania, & Courtney, 2009) successfully instituted a traveling journal club to introduce ambulatory nurses to EBP by creating posters outlining the critical appraisal of evidence related to a topic of interest and circulating these posters throughout various clinics for several weeks at a time. One limitation of this method—nurses had no opportunity for formal discussion of the article. However, the researchers pointed out that subjects reported the presence of informal discussion of the article and the critical appraisal as outlined in these posters. Other creative approaches to adapting journal clubs to the workflow of ambulatory nurses include a breakfast journal club before the clinic opens or lunchtime journal clubs that allow for participation by ambulatory and inpatient nurses.

Multimodal Learning Activities

Growth and development of EBP competencies does not lend itself well to a one-size-fits-all learning strategy. The diversity of roles and experiences of nurse learners, as well as the complex and dynamic nature of the environments in which they practice, presents a challenge to nurse educators. Those educators have developed a variety of novel formats to instill EBP competencies in the nursing workforce to support exemplary professional practice. Introductions to EBP concepts and skills through independent study self-learning packets or e-learning modules and opportunities to practice EBP skills through interactive workshops and train-the-trainer activities help to prepare the nurse for participation in an actual EBP project at the unit or departmental level.

Pierson and Schuelke (2009) piloted an independent study packet (including readings, a hands-on electronic literature search, a written policy review activity, and a post-learning application exercise) supplemented with one-on-one mentoring in strengthening the use of EBP. Based on the positive results of the study, they concluded that "nursing leaders and educators need to provide repetition of learning content and skill acquisition and development of EBP skills to ensure enculturation and sustainability" (Pierson & Schuelke, 2009, p. 175). These investigators clearly understood that EBP workshops alone are not sufficient to build these skills, but that ongoing learning activities need to be available to nurses to grow and sustain EBP competencies.

Although the terms *mentor* and *coach* are often used interchangeably, they are very different concepts. Mentors give advice and teach; coaches facilitate learning or achievement (Fielden, Davidson & Sutherland, 2009). Using nurses with advanced competencies in EBP in both roles can be beneficial in advancing EBP expertise in an organization. Organizations have found the collaboration of nurses in these complementary roles to be successful in increasing EBP skills and knowledge in front-line nurses. Nurses from a large midwestern academic center describe the use of nurse staff development specialists who perform coaching functions in combination with nurse faculty from a variety of academic settings as part-time mentors to facilitate the use of EBP and the development of EBP competencies (Jeffers, Robinson, Luxner, & Redding, 2008).

Having nursing staff members attending educational symposia, workshops, or academies represents another way to inculcate EBP competencies. Program content for clinical skills workshops and other educational venues that incorporate EBP competencies into their curricula ensures that nurses within the organization see EBP in action.

Case in Point

Learning EPB at the Neuro Academy

The Johns Hopkins Nursing Neuro Academy is a three-day program designed to provide both a clinical and professional development opportunity for nursing staff with two years or greater experience in neurosciences. The program content includes a variety of advanced clinical topics in neurosciences, such as deep-brain stimulation, acute spinal-cord dysfunction, or care of families in crisis. A full day-and-a-half of the program is devoted to the development of EBP knowledge and skills. This portion of the program provides nursing staff with a foundation in EBP, a key Magnet tenet.

The program has the following goals:

1. Increase clinical knowledge and skills in neuroscience nursing.

2. Provide mid-level nursing staff with the knowledge to perform EBP.

3. Allow nursing staff to refine their EBP skills by participating in an actual EBP project.

4. Provide an opportunity for staff to contribute to the body of neuroscience knowledge by examining an EBP question that is of importance within the department.

5. Enable staff to apply the EBP process and to serve as leaders for future projects that arise on their unit.

EBP Question

The EBP portion of the Neuro Academy provides participants with an opportunity to learn EBP core competencies while being guided through the process by course instructors serving as mentors. On day one, staff members participate in classes that cover the definition of EBP, why it is important, the EBP process, how to develop an EBP question, and how to appraise various types of evidence. Course content also provides participants with strategies for reading research articles and an opportunity for practice using a sample article. Following the didactic portion of the program, the participants brainstorm a list of clinical questions that concern their practice areas. The group comes to consensus on the question of greatest concern and most relevant to both the neuroscience critical care and the acute inpatient units. A program goal is to make a contribution to the department by way of a practice change or protocol revision based on evidence. Under the guidance of the course instructors, the group then uses the Patient, Intervention, Comparison, and Outcomes (PICO) format to develop and refine their EBP question (Richardson, Wilson, Nishikawa & Hayward, 1995).

The Neuro Academy has formulated a number of EBP questions that have added to the practice of neuroscience nursing, including the following:

-   Will allowing adult craniotomy patients to shower/shampoo their hair 48 hours post-surgery have any adverse consequences to patient outcomes?

-   Is home laundering of scrubs as effective as hospital laundering of scrubs in removing and preventing the transmission of pathogens?

- What are the best practices to prevent errors/accidents related to nurses who are rotating 8- and 12-hour shifts?

- What is the best form of eye care for neurosurgery patients who experience incomplete eye closure to improve patient comfort, eye closure recovery time, and prevention of infection?

EBP Research and Analysis

In the afternoon of day one, participants attend a librarian-led class in the computer lab, where they learn to refine their online searching techniques. Participants use the selected EBP question to conduct an actual literature search. In addition, the group identifies other types of evidence relevant to the EBP question and divides the work of searching between the group members.

Over the next week, class participants search for evidence. Any articles or other types of evidence that are found are submitted to the course instructors. The instructors supply each group member with a complete evidence packet. Participants then read and appraise each piece of evidence in preparation for the next EBP class.

Day two of the EBP program consists of a four-hour session. Generally two weeks pass between day one and day two of the program to allow time for application of day one content of evidence gathering and review. Participants come back together and, as a group, review each piece of evidence for its strength and quality. The group then determines the strength and quality of the evidence as a whole to identify whether or not a change in practice is warranted.

EBP Findings

Organizations have used findings from EBP projects in a number of ways. If sufficient evidence to make a practice change existed, the related protocol was revised. For example, the Neuro Academy found that the closed moisture chamber (lubricant eye ointment and cling wrap) that was currently being used was the most effective method for reducing the incidence of corneal damage in critically ill patients. In this case, the existing practice was validated by evidence and the wording of the standing protocol was modified to clearly reflect the findings. In cases where the evidence was not as strong, the group developed guidelines or informational sheets so that other staff within the department could be informed about the findings.

Career-Altering Event

Participants have consistently rated the Neuro Academy as "excellent," using a "poor" to "excellent" scale. They report that participating in EBP has increased their sense of autonomy and professionalism because they could now influence their practice based on evidence. They report high levels of satisfaction even in making small changes to a protocol or by disseminating information gleaned by the EBP process with fellow colleagues. Kerri Jones who was a nurse-clinician member of the moisture chamber EBP group summed up her experience with the following statement in a written communication to the author. Through the EBP process, "we actually substantiated a task we perform every day with evidence. We could now, with certainty, conclude that the moisture chamber was the best practice. This is a career altering event for me. I came to the realization that every undertaking in my profession, every procedure I perform with a patient comes from more than an order written on a chart. A sense of accomplishment comes to me every time I review the post-op protocol and see the moisture chamber addition."

Structures to Support New Knowledge Generation, Innovation, and Improvement

Because of the constantly evolving nature of the systems and processes of care, nurses have an ethical and professional obligation to contribute new knowledge, innovations, and improvements to patient care, the organization, and the profession (Wolf, Triolo & Ponte, 2008). Not only are nurses compelled to apply new evidence to guide practice, they are also invited to make visible contributions to the art and science of nursing. A multimodal approach is required for this complex endeavor.

EBP Steering Committee

The task of infusing EBP competencies in the nursing workforce is greatly enhanced by the use of an organization-level EBP Committee to facilitate clinical scholarship. The work of this committee is to lead and coordinate the many diverse strategies directed at developing and sustaining EBP competence in nurses. Mohide and Coker (2005) outline action-oriented principles that emerge through the work of such a steering committee:

- Organizational endorsement is critical to ensure development of EBP competence.

- EBP competence

  - Is strengthened through partnerships with academic nurses.

  - Traverses diverse nursing roles, including front-line nurses, thus increasing credibility.

  - Encourages communication with interdisciplinary partners and facilitates nursing influence in organizational decision making.

  - Articulates a shared vision and sense of ownership of the profession.

  - When articulated through the selected organizational EBP model, reflects shared understanding and endorsement of the key tenets of EBP.

  - Is facilitated through use of a practical and easy-to-apply EBP model.

- Using an EBP approach as a committee allows modeling of desired behaviors.

- Employing multiple implementation strategies to develop and maintain EBP competencies increases the likelihood of success.

- Recognizing and acknowledging EBP competence instills EBP throughout the organization.

This last principle is critical to engaging nurses and sustaining interest in developing EBP competencies. Public venues that showcase the contributions of nurses that are the outcomes of EBP and other scholarly activities are very effective in communicating exemplary professional practice. Examples include scholarly activities and EBP fellowship programs.

Scholarly Activities

As nurses generate and acquire new knowledge as a result of EBP projects, organizations need to provide opportunities for these nurses to share their expertise. Organizations can do this externally through publications and poster and podium presentations, nursing grand rounds, and other special events. Through the sharing of these projects, the organization showcases its status as a continual learning environment and engages future learners in both the conduct of EBP projects and the presentation of scholarly works to internal and external audiences.

Mentored publication and poster development and presentation workshops can assist in developing competencies needed to effectively communicate the outcomes of EBP projects to internal and external audiences. By offering these workshops to members of EBP teams, the organization facilitates professional development of evidence dissemination competencies as well as external communication of successes.

Using special events such as nurse scholar days and nursing grand rounds to help nurses build competencies in disseminating and communicating EBP outcomes not only increases organizational capacity for EBP but also improves individual competence in presentations and poster development. By celebrating the successes of the many meaningful EBP projects, research studies, and scholarly presentations, the organization showcases the contribution of nurses to the profession and validates that scholarly activities are valued by the leadership. This exposure engages other nurses who participate in EBP projects to watch and learn from their peers. Using a combination of podium presentations in break-out session format and poster viewing sessions provides opportunity to feature presentations and posters that proficient and expert nurses have presented to external audiences at professional workshops and conferences. In addition, organizations can use this format for the advanced beginner and competent nurse to practice newly learned presentation skills.

Another mechanism organizations can use to build capacity for EBP in the service setting involves integrating acknowledgement of EBP work through special awards. Recognition of scholarly publications and nursing innovations in quality, safety, or service often has the beneficial outcome of engaging other nurses to develop the competencies that enable scholarly development through EBP. Grant awards that offer financial support for the conduct of evidence-based quality and safety projects and/or research studies to generate new knowledge provide the opportunity for teams of nurses to apply and practice EBP knowledge and skills.

Fellowship Programs

A number of publications report on use of fellowships to build EBP competencies. The clinical scholar model developed by faculty at The University of Arizona uses a fellowship program to build capacity for EBP by training front-line nurses to serve as mentors (Brewer, Brewer & Schultz, 2009). This model has been successfully employed in a number of academic medical centers as well as community hospitals in partnership with teaching hospitals.

The purpose of an EBP fellowship is to develop advanced evidence-based practice skills in nurses to prepare them to lead EBP initiatives at the unit, departmental, hospital, or health system level. This fellowship can be executed on a full-time or part-time basis and can extend from six months to a year. Fellowships that are shorter in length might not provide sufficient time for the nurse fellow to accomplish educational or project goals.

Nurses selected for EBP fellowships should meet defined eligibility criteria so that they are poised for success. Examples of eligibility criteria are expressed interest in the fellowship program, written statement of support from the unit manager, demonstration of basic computer skills, and previous participation in a unit or departmental EBP project or EBP or research application course(s). Applicants submit evidence of their qualifications for the fellowship, such as a short essay describing their current abilities and skills and how this fellowship can help them achieve their professional goals. A blinded application review by a diverse group of EBP-competent nurse leaders using stated eligibility criteria promotes a fair and impartial selection.

When selecting an EBP fellow, those making the selection need to look for an individual who demonstrates enthusiasm for EBP and openness to learning. Attributes that enable success in the role include flexibility/adaptability, dependability, attention to detail, time management, customer focus, genuine desire to help and assist others in answering EBP questions, and the ability to embrace differences among team members. Working cooperatively with others enables the EBP fellow to capitalize on the strengths of team members to accomplish team goals.

The role of the EBP fellow includes a variety of responsibilities, such as leading departmental EBP teams, scheduling meetings, leading development of the project plan, and completing assigned tasks like literature searches to facilitate the work of the group. Other aspects of the role involve engaging others in EBP projects, educating nurses on EBP principles and practices, assisting leaders in obtaining answers to clinical or administrative questions, and disseminating stories of successes.

Outcomes of EBP fellowship programs are many and varied. First, these programs promote an increase in numbers of successful EBP projects, providing an additional layer of support for EBP teams that might be burdened with time and energy constraints. Second, EBP fellowships increase the fellow's personal EBP knowledge and skills, which can be transferred to his or her colleagues on return to his or her work setting. Third, these programs enable nurses from one clinical area to interface with and learn from nurses and interdisciplinary colleagues from other departments. Finally, and perhaps most importantly, EBP fellowships increase translation of EBP findings into practice by enabling EBP projects to come to successful closure.

Case in Point

Building Competencies Through an EBP Fellowship

As part of the fellowship experience, I had access to an EBP mentor and was given the opportunity to apply and extend my knowledge of the Johns Hopkins Nursing Evidence-Based Practice (JHNEBP) Model to a clinical EBP project. The practice area to which I was assigned housed a specialty in which I had no prior clinical experience. Nurses in that department had no prior experience with the JHNEBP Model. This laid the groundwork for a mutually beneficial relationship. I brought knowledge and skills related to the conduct of an EBP project to the table; they provided clinical expertise.

Early Investment in Professional Development

The first month of the project was dedicated to EBP training sessions that I conducted for the departmental team. This early investment in the professional development of team members (sharing information on how the model works, demonstrating how to critique a variety of article types, and providing step-by-step instructions on how to build an EBP project) proved to be invaluable. A meticulous review of the definitions of unfamiliar terms (such as the distinction between research and nonresearch evidence and common statistical tests), of how to recognize inconsistencies and flaws in evidence, and of how to identify significant findings were foundational to the group's learning experience.

As the EBP process emerged, the group discovered that the best method to manage evidence review and appraisal was for group members to first critique assigned articles on their own, using the standardized tools provided by the JHNEBP Model, and then to review each article as a group. I acted as facilitator and mentor for the group interaction and gave team members the opportunity to gain confidence and competence in their appraisal skills. As their skill level increased, my facilitation became less necessary, and group members independently critiqued articles and presented their findings to the group. Team members became confident that their literature review formed a strong enough foundation to inform the subsequent steps of the model.

Lessons Learned

During the course of the project, as I became more secure in my own EBP competencies, I learned other lessons related to group process and politics. Early in the process we clearly knew we were dealing with a national problem: *What is the best way to clean and decontaminate ophthalmic equipment?* Therefore, we needed to have departmental leadership at the table from the start. The magnitude of the issue necessitated the positional power of nurse leaders to secure institutional buy-in across the health system clinical sites to make the necessary changes as recommended by the literature and by our own lack of standardized practice. If leadership had not been a part of the process from the beginning, they would not have been convinced of the need for the changes we recommended for the translation phase. The beauty of the EBP process is that it clearly showed the need for the comprehensive changes independent of any single group's agenda or preference. Another lesson learned extended to the fellowship program itself. As the EBP fellow, I became briefly embroiled in a controversy over the team's recommendations. Because of my lack of clinical expertise and credibility in this specialized field, I was unable to resolve these problems without soliciting the aid of hospital leadership. The central group that administers the EBP fellowship modified operating procedures for future mentored experiences to include the recommendation that only the clinical experts on the team should communicate directly with national experts regarding the problem being studied.

Tailoring the teaching of the EBP process to the departmental team's mission, vision, and values is still paying dividends to the institution. Members of the original team are now independently conducting EBP projects on other questions of interest in their field. They are building on the competencies gained in their original learning experience with the EBP fellow and their EBP skills are strengthened with each new project they conduct. In terms of my own continued growth, I have led three subsequent EBP projects in my own clinical area, one of which has expanded into a departmental quality-improvement project with national implications.

Structures to Support Outcomes Management

EBP is outcome-focused. Just as the Magnet designation process recognizes that structure and processes are developed to assure good outcomes, so does the EBP process. EBP allows nurse leaders to demonstrate best practice solutions through innovative structures and processes to achieve clinical and/or administrative outcomes related to nursing, the nursing workforce, patients and families, and organizations (Wolf, Triolo & Ponte, 2008). EBP can support outcome management in a number of ways:

- Integration into the preceptor role to build EBP competencies and promote understanding of linkages between evidence and outcomes.

- Use of structured communications to profile outcomes of successful projects.

- Integration into continuous monitoring plans to ensure sustained improvements.

Integrating EBP into the Preceptor Role

As nursing academia has updated its curricula to include EBP knowledge and skills, the service setting is faced with new expectations on the part of incoming nurses. EBP is expected to be a core competency. Incoming nurses have been taught to actively seek out answers to clinical questions from the evidence. Nothing dampens the enthusiasm of an orientee more than asking a relevant clinical question and being told, "That is how we have always done it, and we are not going to change now." Preceptors need to embrace the value of evidence to their practice and validate the value of evidence in their encounters with orientees. Therefore, preceptors need to be as savvy as incoming nurses about EBP processes. Integration of EBP principles and practices in preceptor training sessions can help achieve this end.

After seven years of intensive preceptor development work using an EBP approach, Vermont nurse leaders updated the role of nurse preceptors to include protector, evaluator, educator/coach, role model (leads by example), and socialization and team leader. This model highlighted the importance of critical thinking development, documentation of evidence, and team leading responsibilities (Boyer, 2008). Clearly, integration of EBP into the preceptor role is a win-win proposition.

Inclusion of EBP competencies for the novice nurse in the first 3 months of the nurse's employment sets the stage for a lifetime of learning. Preceptors should seek out teachable moments when instructing the orientee on hospital protocols and observing the orientee engaging in evidence-based practices to relate that these protocols and practices are based on evidence. The preceptor should encourage orientees to ask pertinent clinical questions, and when the answers are not known, the pair should seek out evidence together.

Skills checklists for the orientation period and a first-year evaluation period should contain incremental EBP knowledge and skill expectations to prepare the nurse to participate as a member of EBP teams. Providing new employees with repeated opportunities to practice new learned skills builds a workforce confident enough to ask pertinent clinical questions and seek out evidence-based solutions.

Structured Communications to Profile Outcomes

Regular reports at standing meetings, website profiles, and periodic EBP-focused newsletters or recurring columns in existing newsletters can help to get the word out about improved outcomes as a result of EBP projects. Interviews with members of EBP teams discussing their efforts to translate findings and the outcomes they have achieved can serve to validate that the efforts of EBP teams yield benefits. Sharing of clinical outcomes achieved by the implementation of a new technique or protocol serves to enhance compliance with that protocol.

A number of studies document improvement in outcomes following implementation of evidence-based practices (Gunningberg, Fogelberg-Dahm &Ehrenberg, 2009; Titler, Herr, Brooks, Xie, Ardery, Schilling et al, 2009; Forbes et al., 2008). Reviews of such articles in EBP-focused newsletters or columns can serve to disseminate how evidence-based practices affect patient outcomes and emphasize the importance of the development of evidence-based practice competencies in improving empirical outcomes.

Measuring Success of Professional Development Initiatives

As with any competency-building initiative, organizations need to evaluate whether the goal of increasing knowledge, skill, and experience with respect to the particular area of desired expertise is achieved. Nurse leaders can measure success of EBP competency-development initiatives in a number of ways. These include competency testing, team evaluation methods, and ongoing monitoring of outcome achievement.

Essential attributes of competency in any practice area are the "application of skills in all domains for the practice role, instruction that focuses on specific outcomes or competencies, allowance for increasing levels of competency, accountability of the learner, practice-based learning self-assessment, and individualized learning experiences" (Tilley, 2008). Evidence-based practice, as one domain of the nurse's role, is accomplished through the application of a specific set of skills and knowledge. Specific competencies as defined in this chapter can serve as the basis for competency checklists to enable documentation of the achievement of these skills through focused instruction. These competency checks should be integrated into existing skills checklists for the various levels of nurse development. Nurses should be held accountable for achieving these competencies and should actively seek out opportunities for practice-based learning.

Evaluation of EBP team activities is another method for determining the effective application of EBP knowledge and skills within these teams. This evaluation can take the form of a self-assessment or assessment by a more experienced team leader who serves as a coach for other team members. Evaluation of EBP team activities should include attention to the effectiveness of the EBP team leader, not only with respect to exhibiting advanced EBP competencies, but also relating to strong coaching competencies. Coaching competencies that are particularly effective in helping EBP leaders guide novice team members through the process include being present, purposeful, positive, and reliable; actively listening and asking questions; and sharing perspectives (Kowalski & Casper, 2007).

Finally, organizations need to monitor the outcomes of EBP projects related to competency development. Have findings been translated into practice? Have identified gaps in evidence spawned the development of research projects? What percentage of staff nurses participate meaningfully in EBP projects? How many presentations and publications have been generated out of EBP projects?

Moving Forward

Nurse administrators are faced with a number of barriers to building capacity for EBP professional development. Rapid environmental change, new technologies, knowledge explosions, competing priorities, time and human/financial resource constraints, and perceived lack of relevance to patient care and role responsibilities all present obstacles to developing EBP knowledge and skills in front-line staff. Transformational leadership; structural empowerment; exemplary professional practice; new knowledge, innovations, and improvements; and empirical outcomes serve as enablers for EBP. Organizations that have embodied these Magnet characteristics are going to be at the forefront of eliminating barriers to translation of best practices in patient care, education, and research. Professional development of EBP competencies in nurses practicing in service settings is imperative as nursing meets the complex challenges of recruiting and retaining nurses in the twenty-first century.

References

American Nurses Credentialing Center (ANCC). (2009). Goals of the Magnet program. Retrieved August 16, 2009, from http://www.nursecredentialing.org/Magnet/ProgramOverview/GoalsoftheMagnetProgram.aspx

Benner, P. (1984). *From novice to expert: Excellence and power in clinical nursing practice.* Menlo Park, CA: Addison-Wesley.

Bloom, B., Englehart, M. Furst, E., Hill, W., & Krathwohl, D. (1956). *Taxonomy of educational objectives: The classification of educational goals. Handbook I: Cognitive domain.* New York: Longmans Green.

Boyer, S. A. (2008). Competence and innovation in preceptor development: Updating our programs. *Journal for Nurses in Staff Development, 24*(2), pp. E1–E6.

Brewer, B. B., Brewer, M. A., & Schultz, A. A. (2009). A collaborative approach to building the capacity for research and evidence-based practice in community hospitals. *Nursing Clinics of North America, 44*, pp. 11–25.

Campbell-Fleming, J., Catania, K., & Courtney, L. (2009). Promoting evidence-based practice through a traveling journal club. *Clinical Nurse Specialist, 23*(1), pp. 16–20.

Church, J. A., Baker, P., & Berry, D. M. (2008). Shared governance: A journey with continual mile markers. *Nursing Management, 39*(4): 34, 36, 38 passim.

Deenadayalan, Y., Grimmer-Somers, K., Prior, M., & Kumar, S. (2008). How to run an effective journal club: A systematic review. *Journal of Evaluation in Clinical Practice, 14*(5), pp. 898–910.

Fielden, S. L., Davidson, M., J., & Sutherland, V. J. (2009). Innovations in coaching and mentoring: Implications for nurse leadership development. *Health Services Management Research, 22*(2), pp. 92–99.

Forbes, S. S., Stephen, W. J., Harper, W. L., Loeb, M., Smith, R., Christoffersen, E. P., & McLean, R. F. (2008). Implementation of evidence-based practices for surgical site infection prophylaxis: Results of a pre- and post-intervention study. *Journal of the American College of Surgeons, 207*(3), pp. 336–341.

Gunningberg, L., Fogelberg-Dahm, M., & Ehrenberg, A. (2009). Improved quality and conprehensiveness in nursing documentation of pressure ulcers after implementing an electronic health record in hospital care. *Journal of Clinical Nursing, 18* (11), pp. 1557–1564.

Huston, C. (2008). Preparing nurse leaders for 2020. *Journal of Nurse Management, 16*(8), pp. 905–911.

Institute of Medicine. (2004). *Keeping patients safe: Transforming the work environments of nurses.* Washington, DC: National Academies Press.

Ironside, P. M. (2008). Safeguarding patients through continuing competency. *TheJournal of Continuing Education in Nursing, 39*(2), pp. 92–94.

Jeffers, B. R., Robinson, S., Luxner, K., & Redding, D. (2008). Nursing faculty members as facilitators for evidence-based practice. *Journal for Nurses in Staff Development, 24*(5), pp. E8–E12.

Knol, J. & van Linge, R. (2009). Innovative behavior: The effect of structural and psychological empowerment on nurses. *Journal of Advanced Nursing, 65*(2), pp. 359–370

Kowalski, K., & Casper, C. (2007). The coaching process: An effective tool for professional development. *Nursing Administration Quarterly, 31*(2), pp. 171–179.

Kramer, M. & Schmalenberg, C. (2008). The practice of clinical autonomy in hospitals: 20,000 nurses tell their story. *Critical Care Nurse 28*, pp. 58–71.

Kramer, M., Schmalenberg, C., Maguire, P., Brewer, B. B., Burke, R., Chmielewski, L. et al., (2008). Structures and practices enabling staff nurses to control their practice. *Western Journal of Nursing Research, 30*, pp. 539–559.

Kring, D. L. (2008). Clinical nurse specialist practice domains and evidence-based practice competencies: A matrix of influence. *Clinical Nurse Specialist, 22*(4), pp. 179–183.

Lee, A. G., Boldt, H. C., Golnik, K. C., Arnold, A. C., Oetting, T. A., Beaver, H. A. et al., (2006). Structured journal club as a tool to teach and assess resident competence in practice-based learning and improvement. *Ophthalmology, 113*, pp. 497–500.

Mantzoukas, S. (2008). A review of evidence-based practice, nursing research, and reflection: Leveling the hierarchy. *Journal of Clinical Nursing 17*, pp. 214–223.

Mantzoukas, S. & Watkinson, S. (2007). Review of advanced nursing practice: The international literature and developing generic features. *Journal of Clinical Nursing 16*, pp. 28–37.,

Mohide, E. A. & Coker, E. (2005). Toward clinical scholarship: Promoting evidence-based practice in the clinical setting. *Journal of Professional Nursing, 21*, pp. 372–379.

Moore, S. C. & Hutchison, S. A. (2007). Developing leaders at every level: Accountability and empowerment actualized through shared governance. *The Journal of Nursing Administration, 27*(12), pp. 564–568.

Nedd, N., Nash, M., Galindo-Ciocon, D., & Belgrave, G. (2006). Guided growth intervention from novice to expert through a mentoring program. *Journal of Nursing Care Quality, 21*(1), pp. 20–23.

Newhouse, R. P., Dearholt, S. L., Poe, S. S., Pugh, L. C., & White, K. M. (2007). *Johns Hopkins Nursing Evidence-based practice model and guidelines.* Indianapolis, IN: Sigma Theta Tau International.

Pierson, M. A. & Schuelke, S. A. (2009). Strengthening the use of evidence-based practice: Development of an independent study packet. *The Journal of Continuing Education in Nursing, 400*(4), pp. 171–176.

Richardson, W. S., Wilson, M. C., Nishikawa, J., & Hayward, R. S. (1995). The well-built clinical question: A key to evidence-based decisions. *ACP Journal Club, 123* (3), A12-A13.

Steenbeek, A., Edgecombe, N., Durling, J., LeBlanc, A., Anderson, R., & Bainbridge, R. (2009). Using an interactive journal club to enhance nursing research knowledge acquisition, appraisal, and application. *International Journal of Nursing Education Scholarship, 6*(1), Article 12. .

Tabari-Khomeiran, R., Kiger, A., Parsa-Yekta, Z., & Ahmadi, F. (2007). Competence development among nurses: The process of constant interaction. *The Journal of Continuing Education in Nursing, 38*(5), pp. 211–218.

Thompson, C. J. (2006). Fostering skills for evidence-based practice: The student journal club. *Nurse Education in Practice, 6*, pp. 69–77.

Tilley, S. (2008). Competency in nursing: A concept analysis. *Journal of Continuing Education in Nursing, 39*(2), pp. 58–64, quiz pp. 65–66, 94.

Titler, M. G., Herr, K., Brooks, J. M., Xie, X. J., Ardery G., Schilling, M. L. et al., (2009). Translating research into practice intervention improves management of acute pain in older hip fracture patients. *Health Services Research, 44*(1), pp. 264–287.

Wolf, G., Triolo, P., and Ponte, P. R., (2008). Magnet recognition program: The next generation. *Journal of Nursing Administration, 38*(4), pp. 200-204.

Zuzelo, P., McGoldrick, T. B., Seminara, P., & Karbach, H. (2006). Shared governance and EBP: A logical partnership? *Nursing Management, 37*(6), pp. 45–50.

Building Core Competencies in Nursing Academia

Evidence-based practice (EBP) brings research alive in nursing education (academia). Research becomes not just about a "t-test" or "threats to validity", but about studies related to nursing practice. Do the findings have rigor? Are the results relevant to nursing practice? Is there a study that can answer the clinical question?

As part of the EBP process, students review available research and propose new research for clinical issues that do not have clear practice recommendations. EBP is an exciting thread in curricula that provides a process for students to effectively examine practice questions and ultimately contribute to nursing knowledge.

EBP competencies are integrated through all levels of nursing education. Baccalaureate students learn the EBP basics. Classes include searching electronic databases for nursing literature, critiquing articles, applying the EBP process to specific clinical questions, and differentiating between using EBP for quality and safety or research. As students move on to graduate education, EBP skills are increased with additional exposure to literature identification, critique, and recommendations for clinical care, education, and administration. At the doctoral level, students initiate and conduct research and capstone projects to answer clinical questions. Coursework provides the methodological skills needed for these activities. This chapter illustrates a road map for integrating EBP within baccalaureate, master's, and doctoral education.

AACN Quality Standards

The American Association of Colleges of Nursing (AACN) establishes quality standards for bachelor's- and graduate-degree nursing education and assists deans and directors to implement those standards. In 1986, the AACN established a national taskforce to define the knowledge, skills, and abilities required for graduates of bachelor's degree nursing education programs. These Essentials of Baccalaureate Education for Professional Nursing Practice were the first set of core standards for nursing programs. They were revised in 2008. The Essentials series also includes standards for master's and practice doctorate programs. In addition, AACN has identified quality indicators for research-doctoral programs. Course content in nursing curricula must comply with these essentials that form the basis for accreditation of nursing educational programs. Additionally, the Institute of Medicine (IOM) (2003) and the National Research Council of the National Academies (2005) have called for dramatic restructuring of all health professionals' education that prepares future practitioners for interdisciplinary practice with information systems, quality improvement, evidence-based practice, and patient safety expertise.

Core Competencies for Baccalaureate Education

Integrating EBP into the baccalaureate curriculum provides students with lifelong learning tools. At the Johns Hopkins University School of Nursing (JHUSON), EBP is a thread incorporated into every course in the four-semester baccalaureate program. Students are guided through the process of locating, reading, evaluating, and applying quality evidence as a basis for nursing practice. Though the overall goal is to prepare nurse generalists, project choices can assist students in further defining their areas of clinical interest. EBP provides a forum for debate on practice issues, with current research serving as the basis for the discussions.

EBP is the focus of AACN's *Essential III* (p. 3), "Professional nursing practice is grounded in the translation of current evidence into one's practice." This standard is exciting and forward-thinking (Table 5.1). Content ranges from models of EBP to collecting and disseminating information. To achieve this Essential, EBP is incorporated throughout the baccalaureate curriculum, including collaboration with service settings.

Table 5.1: AACN Essentials for Baccalaureate Education (2008)

The baccalaureate program prepares the graduate to do the following:

1. Explain the interrelationships among theory, practice, and research.
2. Demonstrate an understanding of the basic elements of the research process and models for applying evidence to clinical practice.
3. Advocate for the protection of human subjects in the conduct of research.
4. Evaluate the credibility of sources of information, including but not limited to databases and Internet resources.
5. Participate in the process of retrieval, appraisal, and synthesis of evidence in collaboration with other members of the health care team to improve patient outcomes.
6. Integrate evidence, clinical judgment, interprofessional perspectives, and patient preferences in planning, implementing, and evaluating outcomes of care.
7. Collaborate in the collection, documentation, and dissemination of evidence.
8. Acquire an understanding of the process for how nursing and related health care quality and safety measures are developed, validated, and endorsed.
9. Describe mechanisms to resolve identified practice discrepancies between identified standards and practice that might adversely impact patient outcomes.

Clinical Practice Questions

At JHUSON, the skills to initiate an EBP project are introduced in the first semester during the nursing trends class. A class presentation covers the basics of EBP with exercises to create clinical practice questions. The PICO format (Patient, Intervention, Comparison, and Outcomes) is used (Richardson, Wilson, Nishikawa, & Hayward, 1995). In this semester, one group project is to complete a scholarly poster presentation of an EBP question. Each group selects an EBP question (see Table 5.2).

Table 5.2: Sample EBP Questions

Aging

What are effective management strategies for constipation prevention in older adults?

What are effective strategies to prevent pressure ulcers in senior citizens?

Obstetrics

What is the pain-medication effect of a doula with laboring mothers?

What is the effectiveness of Kangaroo care in helping premature newborns regulate their respiratory and heart rates?

Adult health

What is the reliability of colorimetric carbon dioxide detection or capnometry as a method to validate nasogastric tube placement?

Does sterile or nonsterile technique make a difference in wound healing in the postoperative wound care of patients with open surgical wounds?

What is the recommended vital sign frequency requirement for patients who are receiving a blood transfusion?

Pediatrics

Is preoperative fasting needed for children prior to surgery?

What is the evidence for the use of complementary and alternative medicine strategies to relieve postoperative pain in pediatric patients?

Psychiatric

What is the best approach to prevent obesity in adult psychiatric patients?

Nursing Administration

What is the best available evidence regarding preventive strategies of sharp and needle-stick injuries?

Does double-check verification of medications prior to administration decrease medication errors?

These EBP questions are based on clinical problems identified by local hospitals and include common clinical problems. Working in groups, students use the PICO format to further define the clinical question. With assistance of the librarian, students conduct a literature search using electronic databases. The question is defined with more precision after searching in established databases such as the Cochrane Database of Systematic Reviews, Agency for Healthcare Research and Quality (AHRQ), Joanna Briggs Institute, Cumulative Index to Nursing and Allied Health Literature (CINAHL), and other databases. Librarian assistance is an important resource to utilize early and frequently in nursing education. Each student reviews and rates two articles for the project. Students summarize their findings in a scholarly poster format. This project provides experience in problem identification, literature search for answers, and clinical decisions based on best evidence. This process continues throughout the remaining courses.

Incorporation of Best Evidence into Care Plans

Second semester clinical courses focus on clinical skills and nursing care plans, requiring the incorporation of best evidence. Students are expected to be knowledgeable of EBP and use the best available evidence for their nursing care plans. The didactic section of clinical courses stresses the best evidence or lack of evidence around specific topics. For example, rigorous evaluation of parent-centered care on a pediatric unit has not been done. Students interested in this topic developed a PICO question and searched for evidence. This emphasis on EBP in the clinical courses sparks interest in students to consider the importance of nursing research in their practice and career goals.

Nursing Research

The third semester includes clinical courses and a three-credit nursing research course. In the nursing research course, students have an option to collaborate with EBP committees at local clinical facilities and participate in the unit's EBP projects. Students are expected to complete the process and make their recommendations for implementation of the evidence. Upon completion of the nursing research course, students can then apply the JHNEBP Model to a selected clinical problem. The course also includes methodological content to insure that students have the tools and skills to evaluate research studies. It provides students with additional opportunity to practice acquired knowledge and skills by creating or selecting an EBP question, using the JHNEBP Model and working in groups of five or six students (Table 5.3).

Table 5.3: EBP Guidelines

Purposes of the EBP Project

The overall purpose of the EBP project is to give students the opportunity to build upon their research-critiquing skills by *identifying and researching a clinical issue and developing practice recommendations* for the issue. Working in a group allows students to learn how research teams divide their work, communicate within and outside the group, and collaborate with other team members. The project also gives students an opportunity to perform an *in-depth exploration of a nursing area of personal interest.*

Description of the EBP Project

The student group either selects a research question from the list provided by clinical nurses or develops their own research question. Each group member is required to locate, critique, and summarize one or two articles. If the group selects a nurse-designed question, the students agree to share their finding with the clinical nurse. In return, the clinical nurse agrees to consult with the student group.

The student group has these responsibilities:

- Searching the literature to obtain recent articles
- Highlighting and critiquing the selected articles
- Summarizing the key findings from the articles
- Making clinical practice recommendations about the topic
- Recording key findings and practice recommendations
- Presenting these findings to the research class and nursing unit

---

Partnering with local clinical facilities provides a win-win experience for students and the clinical facility. Students immediately appreciate the application of EBP to their nursing practice. The student's work is appreciated and used by units participating in this collaboration. Students learn about relevant EBP questions and their work is used beyond the classroom. Nurses in the workforce hear the student's perspective and questions about the practice issue. This dialogue further refines the EBP question. Nursing units also benefit from additional support for their EBP efforts.

Students are directed to search established databases, but they do not always find the answer. For example, one EBP question from The Johns Hopkins Hospital (JHH) is, "What criteria or factors predispose patients to injury post-fall?" This question goes beyond fall-risk assessment. Do any studies assessing risk for injury exist? The students discussed the project extensively with the JHH nurse to understand the question. This process was exciting for students and provided some evidence for the JHH staff to consider an injury-risk scale as an adjunct to the fall-risk scale. Upon completion of the review, the JHH staff might tailor preventive interventions to the specific risk. One student was so interested in the topic that he became a part-time research assistant for a study that grew out of this project. After passing registered nursing boards, he continues to supplement his work as a full-time staff nurse with a part-time job as a research assistant for this study.

EBP also provides an opportunity for faculty to collaborate and provide consultation with clinical agencies. Faculty can provide consultation and training to expand the EBP capabilities of an agency.

Case in Point

Academic-Clinical Collaboration Promotes Unit EBP

Collaboration with service agencies can be initiated by School of Nursing (SON) faculty or a clinical agency. One faculty member provides clinical instruction at a local pediatric specialty hospital, Kennedy Krieger Institute (KKI), and teaches baccalaureate nursing research. As a result of this clinical work, the KKI clinical specialist collaborated with SON faculty to initiate an EBP approach to clinical questions.

Evidence-based practice is the basis of policy and procedures at KKI; however, no formalized EBP process is in place there. KKI is dedicated to helping children and adolescents with disorders of the brain, spinal cord, and musculoskeletal system achieve their potential and participate as fully as possible in family, school, and community life (http://www.kennedykrieger.org). The nursing staff is a vital part of the interdisciplinary team of professionals that assists the patient and family to optimize wellness, prevent further disabilities, and, as needed, adapt to a changed lifestyle. Nurses assist with pre-admission assessment, evaluation and treatment, and discharge planning for patients seen in the inpatient unit and outpatient clinics.

EBP Training Session

The KKI clinical specialist was invited to a one-day JHNEBP education program to launch this initiative. This EBP training session provided insight and direction on how to conduct a systematic review of the literature and use published studies to apply new findings to current clinical practice. The training session also gave direction on how to use EBP to validate policies and procedures by illustrating current clinical practice at other health care facilities. The EBP education program, along with ongoing assistance from the JHUSON faculty member, provided nursing staff with the tools needed to question current clinical practice, explore existing evidence, and, if applicable, translate this evidence into clinical practice. This process allowed nursing staff to dispel any remaining doubts as to whether or not current clinical practice was up-to-date and gave credence to any policy and procedure updates. The clinical agency's lack of experience and/or system for EBP was a potential barrier. However, the willingness to learn and use resources overcame this barrier. The agency used the EBP process taught to the nursing students to increase the knowledge, skill, and experience with EBP in its nursing staff.

At the direction of the KKI clinical specialist, staff nurses were invited to identify clinical practice concerns. A number of questions of particular interest to staff nurses were identified for collaboration with nursing students. The clinical specialist discussed the nursing staff's concerns and the clinical impact of these concerns with the nursing students. One question that arose from this exercise was, "Does negative pressure wound therapy decrease the healing time for stage III and IV decubitus ulcers, and is there a cost benefit?" This question was formulated after several staff nurses questioned whether negative pressure wound therapy was worth the extra time and effort (negative pressure wound therapy dressing changes often take more time compared to traditional moist gauze dressings) and extra cost (negative pressure wound therapy dressing sponges cost more compared to traditional gauze dressings).

The nursing students agreed that this was a question of interest to them and followed the JHNEBP Model to answer the research question. Articles reviewed primarily addressed the adult population and supported the use of negative pressure wound therapy in decreasing the healing time of chronic wounds when compared to traditional moist gauze dressings. The literature also revealed that in the adult population this method decreases the patient's pain because of less frequent need for dressing changes (every 2 to 3 days for negative pressure wound therapy compared to daily for moist gauze dressings); decreases the amount of time dedicated to dressing changes (every 2 to 3 days for negative pressure wound therapy compared to daily for moist gauze dressings); and reduces hospital length-of-stay cost (faster wound healing results in shorter hospital stay).

Mutual Benefit

The nursing students' findings had significant implications to the clinical practice at KKI. Despite the lack of studies in the pediatric population, the knowledge that research existed to support the use of negative pressure wound therapy over traditional moist gauze dressings was very beneficial. The nursing staff members were pleased to learn that although initially the negative pressure wound therapy dressing changes took longer and were more costly, the overall benefit to the patient (decreased healing time, less pain, less frequent dressing changes, and less hospital days) was well worth it. The evidence provided validation for the staff nurses that they were employing the best possible clinical practice for their patients. They identified the lack of data on pediatric patient population as an area of future research.

The nursing students appreciated that their project had relevance for staff nurses that continued beyond the student's receipt of a course grade. The partnership between the SON and the agency was mutually beneficial. Discussions with the clinical specialist, who had been trained in the EBP model used by the students, assisted students in developing a relevant question. At the same time, the agency benefited from the students' evidence search, analysis, and synthesis, allowing nurses to concentrate on translation decisions. A continuing challenge for faculty who desire to build EBP skills in nursing students is to forge relationships with nurse leaders in the community and to assist with skill building of their nursing staff when indicated. In this way, the collaboration will be successful in achieving the goals of both service and academia.

Integration of EBP

In their fourth and final semester, baccalaureate students have an option to choose a course in their clinical area of interest. The adult and child health special topic courses require use of an EBP format to answer a clinical question or perform review of an existing policy/procedure at JHH. These courses embrace the integration of EBP as delineated in the AACN *Essentials* document. EBP utilization is a basic skill required for each new graduate. Novice nurses report feeling more adequately prepared when their nursing programs included a focus on EBP (Li & Kenward, 2006).

Core Competencies for Master's Degree Education

The Essentials of Master's Education for Advanced Practice Nursing was developed by the AACN in 1996. A new task force was appointed by the AACN in September 2008 to revise *The Essentials* and delineate the essential professional competencies that should be acquired upon graduation from a master's degree program in nursing for today's practice. Likely the new version will not be ready by the time this book is published because the task force's timeline is to complete its charge for review and potential approval by the AACN Board of Directors at their July 2010 board meeting and approval by their membership at the October 2010 semiannual meeting.

The current *Essentials* document includes seven foundational standards; Essential I is *Research*. This Essential states that "the goal of the research component of the curriculum should be to prepare a clinician who is proficient at the utilization of research including the evaluation of research, problem identification within the clinical setting, awareness of practice outcomes, and the clinical application of research" (AACN, 1996, p. 6). The competencies for the Research Essential further state that coursework should provide graduates with the knowledge and skills to do the following:

1. Access current and relevant data needed to answer questions identified in one's nursing practice.

2. Utilize new knowledge to analyze the outcomes of nursing interventions, to initiate change, and to improve practice.

3. Use computer hardware and appropriate software and understand statistics and research methods.

4. Utilize information systems for the storage and retrieval of data, consistent with the particular population focus.

5. Initiate a line of inquiry into comprehensive databases to utilize available research in the practice of nursing.

6. Write and communicate effectively—identify a clinical problem, demonstrate an understanding of the research related to this problem, critically analyze the problem and current knowledge, and develop a strategy for the incorporation of the research into the treatment regimen.

In summary, this *Essentials* document delineates the EBP process expectations for master's graduates, which include the ability to identify a practice problem, develop a problem statement, critically review and appraise the relevant evidence, and synthesize the findings for application to practice. In addition, master's students should begin to develop leadership skills and strategies to translate applicable research findings into their practices.

Master's degree programs also use educational standards from specialty organizations—such as the National Organization of Nurse Practitioner Faculties, the American Organization of Nurse Executives, and the National Association of Clinical Nurse Specialists to name a few—to further develop their curricula. These organizations have each developed core and specialty competencies for graduates in the role and population focus specialty, and they all include evidence-based practice competencies.

EBP in the Master's Degree Curriculum

EBP knowledge, skills, and application principles are found throughout the master's program curricula at JHUSON. Two of the master's core courses, Intermediate Biostatistics and Application of Research to Practice, provide content directly applicable to the EBP process. The Intermediate Biostatistics course teaches both the assumptions and theory behind the statistical methods as well as application of their use through problem sets and use of statistical applications. This course is required to be taken prior to the Application of Research to Practice course so that a foundation of statistical understanding is assured. Application of Research to Practice is designed to discuss research methods and designs as they apply to evidence critique and appraisal.

Application of Research to Practice

The course overview describes Application of Research to Practice as follows:

This course prepares students for clinical, management, or education leadership roles in health care through translation of the best available evidence into practice within organizations and application of research for nursing practice. Students will develop skills and knowledge needed to review and synthesize the strength of evidence available, and recommend practice changes if indicated. Topics covered include a review of the research process (including theoretical framework, design, and analysis, and research design hierarchy), research critique, rating and synthesizing the strength of evidence, decision making for practice, research and research translation opportunities (outcomes, evaluation research, quality improvement, cost-effectiveness analysis), risk adjustment, measurement, research ethics and organizational change. (NR110.503 Research Application to Practice, Fall 2009 syllabus)

Course Objectives

The course objectives state that upon completion of the course, the student will be able to do the following:

1. Apply knowledge from the sciences to the advanced practice of nursing through utilization of an evidence-based practice model to answer a clinical, administrative, or education nursing question.

2. Demonstrate advanced skills and expertise in nursing practice through

    a. Critique of research and nonresearch evidence through the knowledge of the research process and the elements of a critique.

    b. Differentiation among designs for nursing research in terms of principles, variables, validity, sampling, procedures, strengths, and limitations, and identifying the gaps in knowledge.

    c. Analysis of various approaches to the measurement of variables and collection of data.

    d. Discussion of statistical methods used for the analysis of research data.

3. Apply management skills to improve services in health care systems by synthesizing the current available evidence on a specific problem and recommending practice changes based on the best available evidence.

4. Analyze the influences of social and health policy on health care delivery and clinical practice through the review of influences on evidence-based practice such as regulation, accreditation, or high priorities for research.

5. Utilize the research process to address problems within areas of advanced clinical nursing practice and nursing systems by synthesiz-

ing the state of knowledge on a specific topic and recommending strategies to test interventions for improvement.

6. Demonstrate ethical decision making in advanced practice nursing by identifying issues in the protection of human subjects enrolled in research, differentiating between quality improvement and research, and discussing the role of the Institutional Review Board in research and quality improvement.

7. Demonstrate cultural competence in advanced practice nursing through discussion of disparities in research and inclusion and exclusion of priority populations.

8. Contribute to the advancement of the nursing profession through

   a. Demonstration of an understanding of the role of advanced practice nurses in leading the use and conduct of research and research methods.

   b. Identification of a gap in knowledge specific to the student's expertise, and recommendations for research and practice based on the identified gaps.

Course Requirements

Among many course requirements, two specifically focus on EBP skills and knowledge. The individual research critique requires the student to demonstrate the ability to critically evaluate a scientific paper in the field of nursing based on the knowledge of the research process and the elements of a critique obtained from the class. For this assignment, the student is required to read and critique an article given by the instructor. The critique includes

- Description of the study design, including strengths and weaknesses

- Identification of the research question or hypothesis with supporting evidence

- Authors' conclusions regarding the research question/hypothesis

- Level of student agreement with article conclusions

- Determination of whether the article effectively answered the research question

Proposed follow-up, for example, a research study, to support translation of research findings into practice

The second key and major assignment of the course is the state-of-the-science paper. The state-of-the-science paper is designed to reflect the student's ability to evaluate and synthesize current and relevant data providing the state of evidence on a specific nursing issue. The assignment requires the student to critically appraise the current evidence on the identified nursing issue, summarize that evidence, and develop a plan to implement evidence-based recommendations from the evidence review (Table 5.4). The paper is submitted in two parts so that students can receive feedback on their definition of the clinical problem, assuring that the actual evidence review is strong and focused.

Table 5.4: State-of-the-Science Paper Guidelines

Part I (5-page limit, excluding title page and abstract):

1. Title page and abstract
2. Problem statement
3. Purpose of the paper
4. Introduction—presents a case for the need to study the topic and its importance to nursing
5. The search strategy, keywords, inclusion criteria, and number and types of evidence reviewed

Part II (10-page limit, excluding abstract, references, and appendices)

1. Abstract—with conclusion added related to the state of the science.
2. State-of-the-science on the nursing issue is described with sources of evidence critically reviewed and synthesized. The evidence is summarized in the JHNEBP Individual Evidence Summary Table format (in appendix).
3. The strengths and limitations of the current evidence are described and the evidence base for practice change is clearly supported or the identified gap in evidence is compelling and significant.
4. Recommendations for translating evidence to practice or initiation of further research are identified and linked to the level of evidence from the above synthesis of literature. These recommendations should include a feasible plan for implementation of EBP, identification of key stakeholders and appropriate interdisciplinary team to assemble. Also, a brief plan for outcome analysis is provided, including independent and dependent variables and method of statistical analysis.

These papers are often used by students to develop a manuscript for submission to a professional journal, which is required in most of the master's options.

Clinical Courses

The master's degree clinical courses place an emphasis on review of evidence in the role- and population-focused specialty area. Students are encouraged by their advisors to choose topics for the research state-of-the-science paper that are in these specialty areas. In addition, the clinical practicum experiences include identification, use and evaluation of clinical practice guidelines, standards of care, and practice protocols. The clinical weekly conference often includes discussion of current guidelines for practice, and the students are asked to review and evaluate them for use in their practice environment. The students are also referred to Internet sites where these guidelines for practice can be downloaded to their Palm Pilots for easy access and reference in the clinical setting. However, these resources are also relevant to other master's students, including those in non-clinically–focused majors. For example, the health systems management students could review and evaluate for use recommendations from the IOM third report, *Keeping Patients Safe: Transforming the Work Environment of Nurses* (IOM, 2003).

Case in Point

Academic-Clinical Collaboration in the Master's Degree Program

As part of Strategies in Nursing Management, a required graduate course in the Master of Science in Nursing (MSN) Health Systems Management program at The Johns Hopkins University School of Nursing (JHUSON), graduate students are required to attend a clinical practicum for 6 to 7 hours per week for 14 weeks. Prior to the commencement of this course, graduate students complete a Clinical Practicum Placement Form that provides course faculty with details of each graduate student's overall professional experience with area(s) of specialization and years in each role, current work experience, career goals post-graduation, and preferred area of interest for practicum experience. This information enables faculty to coordinate meaningful clinical practicum experiences in collaboration with a designated preceptor at each service agency based on each graduate student's areas of interest and career goals. Graduate students are also required to complete a negotiated project with a clear leadership/management focus that contributes to the overall quality of service, efficiency, and success of the mission for the practicum setting. The project chosen by the graduate student must be of value to the student's learning experience and the service agency supporting the practicum experience. An example illustrates how this partnership uses EBP to further the goals of the service agency and provide a rich learning experience for the student.

Project and Practice Issue Identification

The assigned clinical practicum experience for the graduate nursing student took place at a northeastern community hospital that was in the process of implementing a computerized provider order management system (CPOM). The CPOM implementation had already been integrated in some areas of the hospital with relative success; however, data collected by the hospital revealed a continued use of verbal/telephone orders despite CPOM implementation and extremely poor overall compliance with signing these verbal/telephone orders within 48 hours. These findings revealed the lack of buy-in of physicians to use the CPOM system. Percentages of handwritten, verbal, and telephone orders remained much higher than those of orders being entered into the CPOM system.

Within the first few weeks of the clinical practicum experience, the graduate student attended numerous leadership meetings. The meetings were held in response to a growing concern about the lack of the CPOM buy-in and findings that verbal orders were not being authenticated within the 48-hour time frame specified by law and regulation. These regulations surround an important Joint Commission Hospital Accreditation Program Standard, Record of Care, particularly Standard RC.02.03.07 (The Joint Commission, 2009). Armed with master's-level EBP competencies, the graduate student identified a very relevant practice issue. This identification provided an opportunity to conduct an EBP project to critically appraise existing literature to determine proven best practices and strategies that would address the service agency's practice issue. This EBP project had a clear leadership focus that contributed to the overall quality of service, efficiency, and success of the mission for the hosting service agency.

Core Competencies for Master's Education

During the course of gathering data and completing this project to answer the EBP question of mutual interest, the graduate student was prepared to utilize competencies obtained throughout the MSN program of study as delineated by the American Association of Colleges of Nursing (AACN) for achieving core competencies through the EBP process (AACN, 2006). The student conducted a search of published literature using PubMed and CINAHL databases and selected articles that addressed the EBP question for further review. After further review of the published articles, only 15 met the criteria for inclusion in this project. The student used systematic methods and evidence-appraisal tools to critically appraise these articles to identify best practices and strategies implemented at other service agencies to determine the best evidence available that supported and addressed the current practice issue.

A copy of the completed EBP project was submitted to the student's clinical practicum preceptor. The EBP Overall Evidence Summation contained findings and practice recommendations that were presented to nursing leadership. Nursing leadership used EBP findings to validate the plan of action and to improve the overall implementation strategy.

Outcomes/Measuring Success

Leadership submitted a periodic performance review to The Joint Commission regarding Standard RC.02.03.07. They reported the organization's overall compliance with signing of verbal orders within 48 hours. In addition to the reporting of these findings, they also submitted a plan of action to address the organization's compliance. The EBP project completed for this service agency by the graduate student was a success because the findings served as a validation tool for leadership that the planned strategies for the continued CPOM implementation and verbal order signage were in fact evidenced-based. In addition, recommendations outlined in the EBP Overall Evidence Summation provided additional strategies that could be employed in the ongoing efforts to increase compliance with the signing of verbal orders within 48 hours.

Nurse Practitioner Scholarly Paper

A recent curriculum revision to the nurse practitioner clinical sequence at JHU-SON resulted in the development of a required scholarly paper. This paper is to be developed over three semesters and result in a manuscript for submission to a journal before the end of the program. The purpose of the scholarly paper is to investigate a complex clinical problem that has psychosocial and/or behavioral implications. The student is expected to synthesize and integrate knowledge gained from current and previous master's-level coursework and apply this knowledge to a clinical problem by using the best available scientific evidence. The focus of the paper is on nurse practitioner counseling for behavioral change (see Table 5.5).

Table 5.5: Suggested Topics for Nurse Practitioner Scholarly Paper

- Obesity
- Smoking
- Alcohol abuse
- Depression
- Anxiety disorders (general, seasonal affective disorder, panic)
- Chronic pain
- Chronic fatigue
- Insomnia
- Eating disorders

In the first course, the student identifies the problem; begins to review the literature; submits a problem statement in the PICO format; and critically appraises one relevant article from the review. To show integration within the curriculum, nurse practitioner faculty in the next semester require that the student develop the state-of-the-science paper for the Application of Research to Practice course on the topic chosen in the first clinical course. In the final clinical course, the student identifies a journal, provides rationale for journal choice, and develops a manuscript to submit to the chosen journal. It is too early to evaluate this change; however, faculty is encouraged with the development of the manuscript and feels that faculty input throughout the process can increase the manuscript acceptance rate.

Core Competencies for Doctor of Nursing Practice

The Essentials of Doctoral Education for Advanced Nursing Practice (AACN, 2006) outlines and defines the eight foundational standards for the Doctor of Nursing Practice (DNP) curricula and provides some introductory comments on specialty competencies/content. The specialized content, as defined by specialty organizations, complements the areas of core content defined by the *Essentials*. The *Essentials* document *Essential III: Clinical Scholarship and Analytical Methods for Evidence-Based Practice* lists seven competencies to achieve this skill level, including that the DNP program prepares the graduate to

1. Use analytic methods to critically appraise existing literature and other evidence to determine and implement the best evidence for practice.

2. Design and implement processes to evaluate outcomes of practice, practice patterns, and systems of care within a practice setting, health care organization, or community against national benchmarks to determine variances in practice outcomes and population trends.

3. Design, direct, and evaluate quality improvement methodologies to promote safe, timely, effective, efficient, equitable, and patient-centered care.

4. Apply relevant findings to develop practice guidelines and improve practice and the practice environment.

5. Use information technology and research methods appropriately to

    a. Collect appropriate and accurate data to generate evidence for nursing practice.

    b. Inform and guide the design of databases that generate meaningful evidence for nursing practice.

    c. Analyze data from practice.

    d. Design evidence-based interventions.

    e. Predict and analyze outcomes.

    f. Examine patterns of behavior and outcomes.Identify gaps in evidence for practice.

    g. Function as a practice specialist/consultant in collaborative knowledge-generating research.

    h. Disseminate findings from evidence-based practice and research to improve health care outcomes (http://www.aacn.nche.edu/DNP/pdf/Essentials.pdf)

In summary, DNP curricula are required to include advanced skills to review evidence, including both scientific and nonscientific; use advanced analytic methods to appraise the strength and quality of the evidence; synthesize the evidence to make practice recommendations; and lead teams to disseminate and translate evidence to improve practice and patient outcomes.

EBP in the Doctor of Nursing Practice Curriculum

Based on the IOM recommendations for restructured health professional education, EBP knowledge skills and translation of evidence into practice strategies are foundational and a thread through most DNP curricula. The JHUSON DNP program is currently a post-master's DNP option only. The program builds on the current master's program content to prepare nurse leaders for EBP in both direct and indirect nursing roles to evaluate evidence, apply research findings in decision making, translate research into practice, and implement viable clinical and organizational innovations to change practice.

In the first semester, DNP students take two courses that integrate content to meet the first program outcome: utilizes clinical scholarship and analytical methods for evidence-based practice. The first course is called Analytic Approaches for Outcomes Management: Individual and Population, and it prepares the student to analyze epidemiological, biostatistical, environmental, and other appropriate data related to individual, aggregate, and population health to improve quality and safety of health care outcomes. The analytic approaches used in this course require the student to analyze and critique the specific methods for analysis used in the literature.

One analytic-approaches exercise requires the student to do the following:

- Perform a statistics critique of an article, focusing on methods (research question, study design, sample size, power analysis, equivalency, instruments used, variables, and statistical tests used)

- Submit a write-up to include strengths and limitation of the methods and findings

- Develop one suggestion for how the analysis could have been improved

The second course integrating methods for EBP is called Nursing Inquiry for Evidence-based Practice and focuses on EBP techniques as a form of nursing inquiry for the doctoral student. The course evaluates the conceptualization, definition, theoretical rationale, and methods of EBP. As part of the course, the students complete a systematic review of the literature on their capstone practice problem, including problem identification, development of a comprehensive search strategy, and critical review, appraisal, and summarization of the evidence.

In the second semester, the DNP students focus on leadership for EBP and translation strategies for organization and system-wide translation of evidence to change practice. Again, two courses integrate the content. The Organizational and Systems Leadership for Quality Care course facilitates understanding of how to lead, advocate, and manage for the application of innovative responses to organizational challenges. Emphasis is placed on the development and evaluation of care delivery approaches. The priority is to meet the needs of targeted patient populations by enhancing accountability for effective and efficient health care, quality improvement, and patient safety. The Translation of Evidence into Practice course focuses on the integration and application of knowledge into practice through theoretical analysis of case studies that present practical challenges to translation of evidence to improve practice and patient care outcomes.

Finally, in the capstone project experience, DNP students must lead a systems-level improvement in their practice area. The experience enhances the student's ability to employ effective communication and collaboration skills to influence health care quality and safety, and negotiate successful change in care delivery processes across a broad spectrum of health care delivery systems. Upon completion of the capstone, the student will demonstrate

1. Advanced clinical judgment, expertise, and specialization in a defined content area

2. Advanced levels of systems thinking and accountability in designing, delivering, and evaluating evidence-based care to improve health care quality, safety, and outcomes

3. Leadership in the development and implementation of patient-driven, institutional, local, state, federal, and/or international health policy in a select content/specialty area

Core Competencies for Doctor of Philosophy in Nursing

No single organization sets standards for accreditation of PhD nursing programs in the United States; however, the AACN plays an important role with nursing PhD education by bringing leaders in doctoral education together to discuss competencies and best practices for PhD curriculum development.

In this spirit, the AACN published a position statement entitled *Indicators of Quality in Research-Focused Doctoral Programs in Nursing* (AACN, 2001). This document recommends a single set of quality indicators for research-focused doctoral programs in nursing, whether the program leads to a PhD or a DNS degree. The document further recommends that PhD programs of study include core and related course content with a distribution between nursing and supporting content consistent with the mission and goals of the program and the student's area of focus and recommends that coursework include

- Historical and philosophical foundations to the development of nursing knowledge

- Existing and evolving substantive nursing knowledge

- Methods and processes of theory/knowledge development

- Research methods and scholarship appropriate to inquiry

AACN currently has a Task Force on the Future of the Research-Focused Doctorate in Nursing that was constituted in October 2008 and charged to identify the essential curriculum elements necessary to prepare graduates for the roles they are going to assume as scientists and/ or academicians and to explore the evolving relationship between the research-focused doctorate and the practice-focused doctorate as they deal with nursing knowledge. Both doctoral degrees have important roles in creating, facilitating, and leading evidence-based practice in nursing today.

EBP in the Doctor of Philosophy Program

The PhD program prepares nurse scholars to conduct original research that advances the theoretical foundation of nursing practice and health care delivery. However, the foundation of an EBP is also important to the PhD program. This fact is obvious in several electives that are offered to PhD students, including Evidence-Based Nursing Practice and Advanced Seminar in Translational Research. These courses focus on research to answer EBP questions.

Collaboration with Service Agencies

Collaboration between schools of nursing and service agencies provides amazing learning opportunities for students. The collaboration between the

JHUSON and JHH has been strengthened by their partnership to develop the JHNEBP Model. SON faculty members attend the EBP steering committee meetings and provide assistance with hospital research projects. As with any successful collaboration, it takes time and commitment to mutual goals. The quality products of student work can benefit an agency. Students learn the reality of evidence-based clinical practice and make a contribution to improving patient care. The hospital needs knowledgeable new graduates whereas the SON seeks meaningful experiences for students. The relationship is synergistic. Students receive the input from clinical experts and clinical experts have the benefit of student enthusiasm and "new" perspective. Newhouse (2007) describes the synergy between practice and academic partnerships in a graduate research course. These partnerships are a win-win situation for clinical or administrative practice and students and can answer important clinical questions. Engelke & Marshburn (2006) report similar opportunities with a collaborative research team of clinical and academic settings. They report that this arrangement bridges the gap between nursing practice and nursing education. EBP can be a strong facilitator of mutually beneficial academia-practice partnerships. Identification of EBP questions expanded from JHH and outpatient center to KKI and local community hospitals.

Overcoming Barriers

Creating successful partnerships must include identifying and addressing potential barriers. Barriers can exist for students and the agency, and these different barriers require different approaches for resolution. Success is interrelated to the commitment of both the agency and students.

The first barrier for students is their knowledge of the EBP process. At the baccalaureate level, nursing skill competence is a competing priority. The balance between skill acquisition and utilization of the best evidence is learned early in one's nursing career. The new student learns the role of a nurse, including utilizing the best evidence for practice. This learning starts with using the EBP process as a base and building additional skills, that is, research methodology and clinical content, as their learning continues. Additional student barriers include student understanding of EBP relevance and its application to practice and lack of knowledge of research process, methodology, and statistics. These barriers can be overcome through collaboration with nursing units and active learning approaches to research and statistical methods.

Faculty barriers include inconsistent identification in class lectures of EBP and the importance of EBP process to nursing practice, which might be a similar barrier in an agency if EBP is not a priority for nursing administration. EBP models vary among faculty and clinical facilities, which can be confusing to students. Regardless of the model used, the fundamental EBP process is similar across models. Time availability can also be a barrier, as faculty and clinical experts must make time to meet with students and discuss the question. Though initial time is increased when working with students on EBP projects, such an approach can save time in the long run (Stone & Rowles, 2007).

Measuring Success

Success measures vary by educational level. For baccalaureate students, success is knowledge and application of EBP to their nursing practice. Master's and doctoral level students are expected to generate state-of-the-science data and answers to clinical questions. At the graduate level, success is often measured as translation and dissemination. Success is also considered by the quality of the EBP projects completed, the utilization of reports by agencies, and the publication of results.

Data on student opinion of the third-semester EBP project for research class is very positive. In 2006 and 2007, 446 baccalaureate students were surveyed about their satisfaction with the research class EBP project. Most students (91%) thought the project was feasible and instructions were clear (88%). One key component of the JHNEBP process is the use of tools for the evaluation of each article and tables to summarize the evidence, which most students found helpful (86%). The EBP project helped students understand the nursing role (82%) in organizational and clinical decision making within health care facilities. Overall, most (81%) are somewhat or very satisfied with the process and somewhat or very satisfied with the outcome (82%). Student comments support these data. Students reported that the project was "fun," a "good learning tool, hands-on experience," the "most useful assignment in program," and "more interesting and informative than I thought it would be." Some negative comments included "really dislike group work," "waste of time," and "hard to critique articles before content covered in class" (Shaefer and Newhouse, 2007).

Evaluation of the agency perspective is an important component of the process. Students are invited to participate in more projects, and the results are very well received. The long-term goal is to expand collaboration and provide assistance to units with student clinical papers (see Special Topics in Nursing sidebar). These can be focused on current questions identified by nursing units. The ultimate goal is to make nursing education relevant while supporting current nursing staff.

Special Topics in Nursing

Introduction to Acute Care of Children Evidenced-Based Practice Paper

Purpose:

The purpose of the evidence-based paper is to provide students the opportunity to apply evidence-based practice analysis skills learned in previous courses. Students identify a practice guideline or practice issue in the pediatric critical care setting and conduct a critique of the literature that supports this practice or guideline. Students are encouraged to identify something of practical interest to both them and a potential future employment setting.

Guidelines:

The topic of the practice guideline includes:

- Practice guideline or issue

- Source of guideline

- Practice setting

- If critiquing a practice guideline, use the guideline's reference list to identify four data-based research articles used to develop the guideline. If articles are greater than five years old, search the literature for more recent articles.

- If critiquing a practice issue, conduct a literature search for four data-based research articles related to this practice.

- Using the JHNEBP Evidence Rating Scale, evaluate the quality of the evidence in the four research articles.

Conclusion

EBP is a crucial component of nursing education. Student competencies vary by educational level. Baccalaureate students learn the EBP process, research methods, and application of EBP to clinical practice. Master's and doctoral student competencies range from state-of-the-science papers to original translational research. All of these skills are essential to assure that nursing practice is based on the best evidence.

References

American Association of Colleges of Nursing. (2008). The essentials of baccalaureate education for professional nursing practice. Retrieved May 21, 2010, from http://www.aacn.nche.edu/education/pdf/BaccEssentials08.pdf

American Association of Colleges of Nursing. (2001). Indicators of quality in reasearch-focused doctoral programs in nursing. Retrieved on May 22, 2010, from http://www.aacn.nche.edu/publications/positions/qualityindicators.htm

American Association of Colleges of Nursing. (1996). The essentials of master's education for advanced practice nursing. Retrieved May 21, 2010, from http://www.aacn.nche.edu/Education/pdf/MasEssentials96.pdf

American Association of Colleges of Nursing. (2006). The essentials of doctoral education for advance nursing practice. Retrieved February 15, 2010, from http://www.aacn.nche.edu/DNP/pdf/Essentials.pdf

Engelke, M. K. & Marshburn, D. M. (2006). Collaborative strategies to enhance research and evidence-based practice. *Journal of Nursing Administration, 36*(3), pp. 131–135.

Institute of Medicine. (2003). *Keeping patients safe: Transforming the work environment of nurses.* Washington, DC: National Academy of Sciences.

The Joint Commission. (2009). *Behavioral health care accreditation program. 2009 chapter: Record of care, treatment, and services.* Retrieved February 15, 2010, from http://www.jointcommission.org/NR/rdonlyres/FF84F337-FEC3-48AE-92A8-ABBD91F70DDF/0/B_RevisedChapter_BHC_RC_20090323v2.pdf

Li, S. & Kenward, K. (2006). A national survey of nursing education and practice of newly licensed nurses. *JONA's Healthcare Law, Ethics, and Regulation, 8*(4), pp. 110–115.

National Research Council of the National Academies. (2005). *Advancing the nation's health needs: NIH research training programs.* Washington, DC: National Academies Press.

Newhouse, R.P. (2007). Collaborative synergy: Practice and academic partnerships in evidence-based practice. *Journal of Nursing Administration, 37*(3), pp. 105–108.

Richardson, W. S., Wilson, M. C., Nishikawa, J., & Hayward, R. S. (1995). The well-built clinical question: A key to evidence-based decisions. *ACP Journal Club, 123*, pp. A12–A13.

Shaefer, S. J. M. & Newhouse, R. P. (2007, November). *Hospital nursing staff and undergraduate nursing students collaboration on evidence-based practice projects.* Paper session presented at the Sigma Theta Tau International 39th Biennial Convention, Baltimore, Maryland.

Stone, C. & Rowles, C. J. (2007). Nursing students can help support evidence-based practice on clinical nursing units. *Journal of Nursing Management, 15*(3), pp. 367–370.

Managing the EBP Project

The Johns Hopkins Nursing Evidence-Based Practice (JHNEBP) Model and Guidelines define a process that nurses can use to conduct evidence-based practice (EBP) projects. The *PET* acronym describes three distinct phases of this multi-step process (*Practice question*, *Evidence*, and *Translation*). Consisting of 18 discrete steps, this process can be daunting to the novice EBP team. Careful project management helps the team stay on track and achieve overall project success. This chapter acquaints the reader with the necessary competencies to effectively manage EBP projects.

Essentials of Project Management

The Project Management Institute (PMI), a world-renowned association for project management professionals, defines a *project* as "a temporary endeavor undertaken to create a unique product, service, or result" (PMI, 2008, p.5). A project has a distinct beginning and end with structured tasks to achieve a well-defined goal. *Project management* is "the process by which projects are defined, planned, monitored, controlled, and delivered such that the agreed upon benefits are realized" (Association for Project Management, 2006, p, 3). Most projects require a focused effort to execute. They are often characterized by uncertainty and complexity. Lack of planning and coordination of effort can result in a waste of precious time and human resources and lead to failure to achieve project goals.

An EBP project is conducted to inform the nurse's practice in whatever setting the nurse provides services. The desired end product, or *deliverable*, of the EBP project is the translation of findings into the nurse's practice. Today's nurse deals with multiple competing priorities. The team needs to manage the EBP project to ensure completion of project tasks and translation of findings. Managing a project requires knowledge and a particular set of skills with which the nurse might be unfamiliar. Mastery of basic project management competencies can help the EBP team meet its goals.

Project Attributes

The first step to effectively manage EBP projects is to become familiar with the primary characteristics of a project. Schwalbe (2007) offers a list of project attributes that can be applied to the EBP project. Each project has a *unique purpose or objective*. An EBP project is designed to answer a specific practice question in a structured, analytic manner.

Projects have a defined life cycle that includes the following processes: initiation, planning, executing, monitoring and controlling, and closing (PMI, 2008). The work of the EBP team is *time-limited* and *temporary* in nature. After the question is answered and findings are translated into practice, the team might disperse, or it might choose to initiate a new EBP project.

The EBP project is developed using *progressive elaboration*. Simply put, the practice question is broadly defined at first, and the team progresses to a clearer definition of specific details as it works through the process of developing the practice question; procuring, analyzing, and synthesizing the evidence; and translating findings.

A project *requires sufficient resources* to accomplish its aims. EBP projects call for commitment of time and energy from team members, organizational infrastructure, and access to credible knowledge sources and mentors. These resources might be required from a single department or discipline or from several different departments or disciplines, depending upon the nature of the practice question, the composition of the EBP team, and the stakeholders involved.

Generally, each project has a primary *sponsor.* Sponsors are people who see a need for change and have the commitment to make it succeed. The sponsor of an EBP project can be an individual nurse, a nursing unit, a group of nurses across multiple units, an interdisciplinary team, or an established committee. For example, a clinical standards committee that is updating a patient care protocol might ask a clinical question to uncover best practices with respect to a particular aspect of care defined in the protocol. Sponsors could also be a group of staff nurses who are looking at the best ways to streamline a particular clinical task without adversely affecting patient outcomes.

Finally, projects involve *uncertainty.* The outcome of an EBP project can take a variety of forms depending upon the strength and quality of evidence related to the practice question. Even when evidence for change is compelling, barriers to translation might exist that present risk and uncertainty.

Project Constraints

Managing projects involves trade-offs. Four major constraints need to be managed to assure success:

- Time

- Human and material resources

- Scope

- Money

Nurse members of the EBP team commit their time and energies, which would have been engaged in other aspects of their practice, to the conduct of the project. Nurse leaders allocate staff time to accomplish project objectives or to assist other nurses in the development of EBP competencies, diverting these resources from other activities for the duration of the project.

Limited resources demand thoughtful definition of the project scope and attention to the financial costs associated with the project. When developing the scope of the project, the team defines the patient or staff populations addressed by the practice question, what type of change is anticipated (for example, new responsibilities, processes, systems, or training) and the location(s) of affected individuals (for example, specific units, departments, or organized groups).

Well-meaning project teams often fall prey to *scope creep*, the subtle increase in or change of project requirements over time. For example, a team might be looking for best practices in managing skin care in orthopedic patients on a particular patient care unit. The original plan might include a pilot test of one or more best practices on orthopedic patients within this setting. During the course of the evidence phase, a team member who uncovers evidence of effective skin care regimens in neurosurgery patients might suggest that the team expand the scope of the question to include skin care on neurosurgery patients. Though this question might be of interest to the team, if the team adds an additional population, the scope of the project and the resources associated with executing the project might increase exponentially. Efficient EBP project management ensures that team members pay attention to containing the scope of the project and the dollars associated with indirect staff time.

Project Management Knowledge Areas

Nurses need to be aware of the basic knowledge areas related to managing projects:

- Human resources

- Communication

- Integration

- Scope

- Time

- Cost

- Quality

- Risk

- Procurement (PMI, 2008)

The specific processes that fall under each knowledge area are well-defined for professional project managers. The EBP team is not expected to master all processes that make up each project management knowledge area. However, particular processes can be of benefit to the team.

Human Resource Management

When setting up an EBP project, a team needs to have an identified project leader. This person takes responsibility for ensuring that the project stays on track, coordinates team-building activities, provides feedback to the team, resolves issues, and coordinates team activities. The project leader can be a nurse with experience doing an EBP project or one who leads the team in a mentored experience.

Projects are more successful if they have the right people on the project team—people who understand their roles and responsibilities, are engaged in the project, and are committed to its completion. Human resource management includes assembling the project team; developing team members' knowledge, skills, and expertise in evidence-based practice and team collaboration competencies; and managing the team for performance.

Team member roles and responsibilities should be clearly defined. This clear definition serves a twofold purpose. First, it ensures that each individual has a clear understanding of the expectations of his or her role as a member of the EBP team. Second, it allows the team leader to monitor and evaluate team performance. EBP project leaders often assign responsibilities to team members based on the members' particular skills and experience level. In learning organizations, team leaders might take a different approach, assigning responsibilities to mentored nurses who need further skill development in the particular area.

When planning for and acquiring an EBP team, the team leader needs to take several factors into consideration. The first factor is *interest*; that is, is the particular problem of interest to the potential team member? The next factor is *availability*. The team leader needs to know who is available to be released from other job responsibilities to participate on the project and when these individuals can be available. A third factor is *ability*. Does the potential team member have the competencies required to complete an EBP project or does that individual need to be mentored? Fourth, has the person had the *experience* of participating on an EBP project in the past? A final factor that a team leader must consider is *allocation of resources*—can the nurse's manager afford to provide time away from front-line patient care activities so that team members can participate?

A people-management worksheet can be helpful in assigning tasks to individuals. It allows for documentation of each team member's role, the authority accompanying the role, skills required to perform the role, and responsibilities accompanying the role. This worksheet allows team members to document and communicate mutually agreed upon expectations of each other so that work is well-coordinated. Table 6.1 is a sample people-management worksheet completed for an EBP project.

Table 6.1: People-Management Worksheet Excerpt

Activity	Required Competencies	Hours Required	Time Frame	Source	Responsible Person (Contact Info)
Curriculum development	Curriculum development, Learning management system use	30 hours	April 2010	Clinical department	Joe (ext. 2222)
Competency checklist development	Skills checklist development	16 hours	May 2010	Pilot unit	Susan (ext. 3333)

Communication Management

A helpful strategy to set the stage for ongoing communication is the kickoff meeting. Identified stakeholders can be invited to hear a project overview, share their communication needs, and endorse the communication plan. The meeting to establish the communication plan should address the following questions:

1. Who needs information—persons or groups?

2. What information do they need—will it have a standard format?

3. When do they need it—how often?

4. Who will provide it—team leader, team member?

5. How will they receive it—face-to-face meeting, e-mail, formal report?

To ensure attention to this critical component, the communication plan should be included in the overall project plan.

Integration Management

Integration management incorporates those activities that allow the team to integrate the various pieces contributed by team members along the course of the project. Though the EBP team does not necessarily need to develop a formal project statement, the team should specify the reason for doing the project, the scope of the practice question, and how the project fits into the larger organizational or unit picture. Many EBP models use the PICO (Patient, Intervention, Comparison, and Outcomes) process to assist in the development of the practice question. This process is fully described in the literature (Newhouse, Dearholt, Poe, Pugh, & White, 2007) and includes specification of how and why the question was identified and the scope of the practice question.

The project management plan is a key deliverable for integration management, and EBP teams benefit greatly from incorporating this process into their work. The project management plan brings together all of the activities planned for the project and "provides a reference document for managing the project" (APM, 2006, p. 5). The EBP team directs and manages the execution of the project plan and then formally ends the project following translation of findings into practice.

Scope Management

The team needs to control what is and what is not within the scope of the project. In the course of searching for and analyzing evidence related to the practice question, the team inevitably encounters many ideas and best practices not directly related to answering the question at hand. Trying to address implementation of all of these practices in the project plan is tempting. Scope creep compromises the team's ability to focus on translating findings that directly relate to the question of interest.

An important tool that outlines the project scope is the Work Breakdown Structure (WBS), which is a graphical representation of the steps involved in accomplishing project aims. The WBS lists all of the project tasks, from general tasks, for example, evidence search, to more detailed sub-tasks, for example, identification of key words and selection of search databases (Kaufman, 2005). The process of constructing a WBS not only forces team members to think about all of the steps required, but also allows them to break the project down into smaller, more manageable steps. It provides the team with a framework on which to base project status monitoring activities. If a step is not part of the WBS, then it is not part of the project. The WBS provides the foundation for the project plan. Figure 6.1 is an example of a WBS developed for the translation phase of an EBP project.

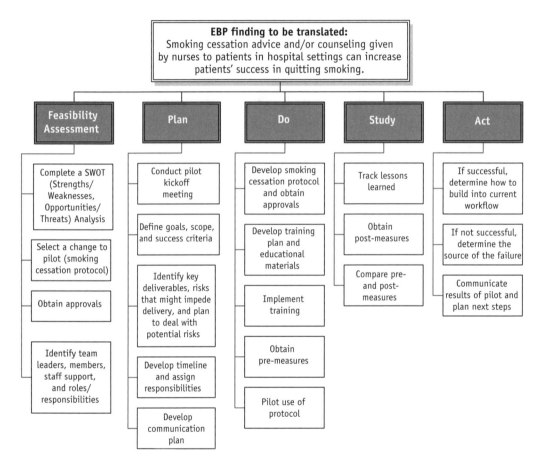

Figure 6.1: Work Breakdown Structure Excerpt

Time Management

After the WBS has been developed and the team has listed required activities, the team can benefit from a structured time management process. During this process, team members sequence activities, determine which activities are dependent on other activities, specify estimated duration of each activity, develop an overall project timeline, and set project milestones. This information is entered into the overall project plan.

Although more sophisticated software like Microsoft Office Project is available to assist in the development of elaborate project timelines and plans, EBP teams can develop a simple Gantt chart in a standard spreadsheet program like Microsoft Excel to plan and schedule projects and to monitor the EBP project's progress over time. A Gantt chart is a classic graphical representation of task duration against time progression that was developed in the early1900s by Henry Laurence Gantt, a management consultant and mechanical engineer (Gantt, 1974).

The team can visualize scheduled and actual progress of planned project activities. Table 6.2 illustrates an example of a Gantt chart for an EBP project. Gray blocks indicate that the activity has been completed on time.

Table 6.2: Gantt Chart Excerpt

Project Activity	Responsibility	Start Date	End Date	Week 1 1/25/10 to 1/29/10	Week 2 2/1/10 to 2/5/10	Week 3 2/8/10 to 2/12/10	Week 4 2/15/10 to 2/19/10	Week 5 2/22/10 to 2/26/10
Identify stakeholders	Team leader	1/25/10	1/29/10					
Conduct stakeholder analysis	Team members	1/25/10	2/5/10					
Secure leadership support	Team leader	1/25/10	1/29/10					
Identify pilot unit	Team members	2/8/10	2/12/10					
Develop action plan for pilot	Team members	2/1/10	2/26/10					

Cost Management

Teams need to not only control costs but also to actively include a budget when planning the EBP project. Though the EBP team might not have a budget for its work, the cost of nurse team members' time on project-related activities and any administrative costs (for example, copying, word processing, and librarian fees) should be estimated and tracked. This information is helpful when accounting for indirect time and supply costs in financial reports. In addition, if translation of findings requires financial resources, teams need to quantify these cost estimates, especially if additional funding is going to be required to proceed with evidence translation. Articulating cost enables the team to present a more comprehensive report to leadership. Table 6.3 provides an excerpt from a budget planning worksheet for an EBP project implementation.

Table 6.3: Budget Planning Worksheet Excerpt

Activity or Item	Cost per Item	# of Items	Total Cost	Supplier	Funding Source	Date Required	Responsible Person
Data collection	$43/hr	1 RN @ 160 hrs	$6880	Nursing unit	Unit operating budget	3/8/2010 through 4/2/2010	Nurse manager
Data analysis	$45/hr	1 RN @ 10 hrs	$450	School of nursing	Grant funds	4/12/2010 through 2/23/2010	Grant administrator

Quality Management

Quality management becomes very important in the translation phase of an EBP project. After making a recommendation for change based on analysis and synthesis of evidence and deciding to implement a change in current structure or processes, the team should begin quality-planning activities. These activities include developing a quality-management plan with appropriate metrics and a determination of baseline performance with respect to these metrics.

Rapid cycle tests of change such as the Plan-Do-Study-Act (PDSA) framework (Lipshutz, Fee, Schell, Campbell, Taylor et al., 2008) are very effective in managing the quality of changes implemented as part of the EBP project. During the *Plan* phase, the EBP team answers *who, what, when, where, how,* and *why* questions related to the evidence-based change and develops an action plan to pilot this change. Measures are selected to allow the team to know whether the change is successful. Baseline performance on these metrics is measured. During the *Do* phase, the change is implemented, and the team monitors for anticipated and unanticipated effects of the change. The team takes the opportunity to *study* the effects of the change during the next phase. Finally, the team makes the decision to fully implement a successful change (*Act*) or to conduct a test of a different evidence-based change if the original change was unsuccessful in achieving desired outcomes.

Quality management ensures that "both the outputs of the project and the processes by which the outputs are delivered meet the required needs of stakeholders" (Association for Project Management, 2006, p. 6). A quality-management worksheet can be helpful to keep track of quality issues that occur in the conduct of the EBP project. This worksheet is often organized in terms of deliverables or outputs, criteria for judging the quality of the process by which the deliverables were obtained, persons responsible for producing the deliverable, and corrective or preventive actions to improve the quality of the deliverable. Table 6.4 provides an excerpt from an EBP quality-management worksheet for the translation phase of an EBP project conducted by school nurses.

Table 6.4: Excerpt from an EBP Quality-Management Worksheet

Deliverable	Quality Criteria	Responsibility	Pass/ Fail	Corrective Action
Education packet on improving family-centered care in schools	Uses competency-based approach Includes pre- and post-test to assess learning	Marie and Peggy	Fail	Consultation with nurse education liaison with expertise in competency-based testing

Risk Management

Risks abound in any project; EBP projects are no exception. A project risk is any potential source of deviation from the project plan (PMI, 2008). Risks are uncertain. Those that have a negative impact on the project are called *threats*; risks that have a positive impact on the project are called *opportunities*. The EBP team needs to identify potential threats and opportunities and analyze these risks in terms of probability of occurrence and impact if they occur. They should make efforts to increase the probability of opportunities and reduce the probability of threats by developing contingency plans to deal with the identified threats. These activities can be formally documented in a risk-management plan.

One tool that is very helpful in terms of quantifying project risks is the SWOT (Strengths-Weaknesses-Opportunities-Threats) analysis. A SWOT analysis enables the team to identify facilitators and barriers when planning all phases of the EBP project, but has particular application to the translation phase. A technique that has been used in strategic, career, and project planning, the SWOT analysis is an effective way of helping the team focus its activities on areas in which it is strongest and where the most opportunities lie (Pearce, 2007). During a SWOT analysis, the EBP team considers its strengths and weaknesses and uses information from these internal factors to capitalize on strong points and develop remedial actions for weak points. The team also recognizes opportunities and threats and uses information from these external factors to recognize opportunities that arise and to deal with threats to project completion. Table 6.5 depicts a sample SWOT analysis conducted by an EBP team whose practice question centered on best practices in documentation of skin assessment to support quality monitoring of pressure ulcer prevention and treatment.

Table 6.5: Sample SWOT Matrix for Pressure Ulcer Prevention EBP Project

Strengths	**Weaknesses**
• EBP project team is led by content experts in pressure ulcer prevention and treatment. • EBP project team has experience in conducting EBP projects and translating findings.	• Staff members on nursing units do not have sufficient expertise in pressure ulcer staging. • Clinical documentation is a hybrid model (part electronic, part paper) and does not prompt nurse to document data related to pressure ulcer screening.
Opportunities	**Threats**
• Organization is moving to a paper-lite documentation system that is mostly electronic and is in the design phase. • Potential to improve documentation of skin and wound using decision support tools. • Increased leadership attention because of changes in Medicare reimbursement for hospital-acquired conditions.	• Nursing staff is challenged by multiple competing priorities. • Electronic documentation rollout is contingent on continued funding and sufficient manpower.

Another tool that is useful for helping to prioritize negative risks is the probability-impact matrix (Ginn & Varner, 2004). The team lists the likely risks that the EBP project faces and assesses the probability of the risk occurring. The team also assesses the size of the negative impact (in terms of organizational or patient outcomes) should the risk occur. This information can be depicted graphically, with probability on the y-axis and impact on the x-axis. Risks are plotted on the chart, with respect to these characteristics and are categorized into one of nine groups based on low, medium, or high probability of occurrence and low, medium, and high impact on the project should the risk occur (Ginn & Varner, 2004).

The team's top priorities should be those risks that fall in the high probability, high impact category. Contingency plans should be developed for these risks and for those in the low probability/high impact group. Figure 6.2 shows a sample probability/risk impact chart for a hypothetical EBP project that resulted in development of a new protocol for preventing pressure ulcers in nursing home residents. In this example, the EBP team wants to be confident that the people and equipment needed for the translation project (wound care specialist, equipment such as mattresses and seat cushions, and aids such as heel protectors) are available in time for implementation and that contingency plans are in place if resource or cost constraints occur.

Assessing the Probability and Impact of Risks

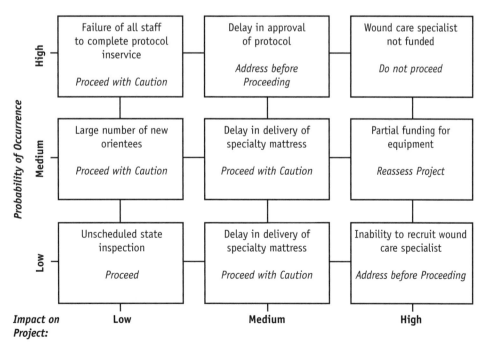

Figure 6.2: Sample Probability/Risk Impact Chart

Procurement Management

For the EBP project, procurement management is a knowledge area that comes into play with the need to purchase or acquire products or services from external sources to accomplish project goals. For example, a community hospital might need to procure online library services from an academic medical institution to support EBP projects. Another example is seen when the team wants to make an evidence-based change in the manner in which wounds are dressed that requires the addition of a new type of dressing material to the supply management system. Though front-line nurses might not be directly involved in purchasing operations, they often have a role in product evaluation and selection decisions. The team should seek assistance from persons who can facilitate the approval, contract negotiation, and procurement process.

Planning an EBP Project

Planning a project requires defining success, identifying the practice question, providing structure, planning artfully, and establishing controls.

Defining Success

Before planning an EBP project, teams need to lay the groundwork for success. First, the team should define what *project success* means. How does the team determine that the project has been successful? Is this conclusion based on team performance against process measures? For example, the team might measure success by its ability to keep to specified scope, time, and cost constraints.

Another measure of success evaluates the outcome of the project, such as the quantity or quality of the deliverables produced. For example, success could be measured by the number of evidence-based practices identified for consideration and implementation by the team, the nursing unit, or the organization as a whole. If practice variations are a safety concern, the team might feel a sense of achievement if it finds one effective practice to standardize across the organization. Success could also be measured by the quality of the deliverables. For example, the team might feel a sense of accomplishment if project findings indicate that the state of the evidence is not sufficiently robust to warrant a change in current practice.

Another measure of success could focus on fulfillment of stakeholders' interests. For example, the team might define success by the level of customer satisfaction with the deliverables produced. First, the team needs a clear understanding of its customers, for example, nurses who are required to institute practice changes based on the evidence or other health care team members whose work might be affected by the changes. Second, the team needs to understand the drivers of satisfaction for each of these customers. Other measures of success include the extent to which team members and other staff learned new EBP competencies and how the EBP project influenced staff attitudes toward EBP.

Defining the Practice Question

In planning for maximal success, the team needs a clear and complete statement of the problem so that it understands how its practice question fits into the larger picture. For example, an EBP team that is trying to find best practices related to fall prevention should be cognizant of the fact that the hospital is in the process of developing a bed replacement plan. In this example, the team might want to narrow the practice question to look at the effectiveness of bed alarms in reducing falls.

The team should identify all internal and external stakeholders. Stakeholders are defined as "persons or organizations … who are actively involved in the project or whose interests may be positively or negatively affected by the performance or completion of the project" (PMI, 2008, p. 23). Knowledge of project requirements and expectations of all stakeholders allows the EBP team to manage the influence of the various stakeholders to ensure project success. For example, during an EBP project probing the best way to assess dyspnea in oncology patients, the EBP team consisting of inpatient nurses might find that nurses in the outpatient oncology clinic are hoping to use whatever tool is selected by the EBP team in their practice. The astute team leader might invite an outpatient nurse to join the EBP team to provide the outpatient nurse with the opportunity to participate in the process so that the outpatient nurse develops skills to conduct a similar project in her own clinical area.

The team should look at a realistic timeline for answering the EBP question. The following temporal factors need to be addressed when developing the timeline: the time commitment of individual team members (when and how often they are available to do project-related activities), anticipated duration of each activity, timeline associated with any external dependencies (for example, completion of a pilot test can be dependent on the delivery of a product purchased from an external source), and time frames or limits associated with available resources (for example, access to meeting rooms might be limited during certain times).

Providing Structure

The next key to planning a successful EBP project is to provide structure. The team needs to understand what it needs to do and how it needs to do it. As previously mentioned, the WBS is a helpful way to outline the various activities required for project completion. The Johns Hopkins Nursing Evidence-Based Practice (JHNEBP) Project Management Tool (Newhouse, Dearholt, Poe, Pugh & White, 2007) outlines the PET (Practice question, Evidence, Translation) process in simple steps so that team members do not have to process all components at once. The WBS starts off broadly defined and becomes more granular as the EBP project unfolds. For example, at the start of the project, the team has not completed the analysis of evidence that leads to a recommendation for change. The specific steps for evidence translation are dependent upon the type of change being piloted.

As part of the project plan, tasks are assigned to team members based on their individual capabilities and developmental needs. Task allocation can be used as a way to capitalize on current knowledge and skills and build new competencies for future projects. Additionally, teams need to order tasks in a reasonable sequence and estimate time involved in the project. PERT (Program Evaluation and Review Technique) charts are helpful tools for managing large, complex projects with a high degree of intertask dependency. This technique involves the following steps as suggested by the Internet Center for Management and Business Administration, Inc, (2009):

1. Identification of specific activities and milestones

2. Determination of proper activity sequence

3. Construction of a network diagram

4. Estimation of time requirements

5. Determination of a critical path

6. Update of the chart with project progression

Figure 6.3 depicts a sample PERT chart for an EBP project.

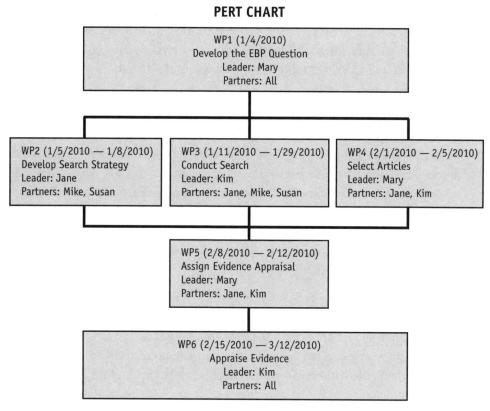

PERT CHART

WP1 (1/4/2010)
Develop the EBP Question
Leader: Mary
Partners: All

WP2 (1/5/2010 — 1/8/2010)
Develop Search Strategy
Leader: Jane
Partners: Mike, Susan

WP3 (1/11/2010 — 1/29/2010)
Conduct Search
Leader: Kim
Partners: Jane, Mike, Susan

WP4 (2/1/2010 — 2/5/2010)
Select Articles
Leader: Mary
Partners: Jane, Kim

WP5 (2/8/2010 — 2/12/2010)
Assign Evidence Appraisal
Leader: Mary
Partners: Jane, Kim

WP6 (2/15/2010 — 3/12/2010)
Appraise Evidence
Leader: Kim
Partners: All

Figure 6.3: Sample PERT Chart

Planning Artfully

The EBP team leader cannot develop the project plan alone; team involvement in planning is critical to its success. Participation in planning enables team members to feel a sense of ownership of the EBP project. The project leader is often responsible for actually putting the formal plan together. However, by contributing information and ideas, the team assists the project leader by making use of all available expertise and ideas.

Another hallmark of a well-thought-out plan is determining the quality of work. Using defined measurable criteria, the team ensures that no step of the process is completed until defined criteria are met. For example, if the project plan calls for a search of six databases for evidence using specific keywords, then the search is not complete until all in the plan is accomplished. The team specifies the search strategy and uses this specification to determine if the search was carried out as planned.

One rule to keep in mind when conducting EBP projects is to do the best job possible, not to be perfect. Competing priorities, time constraints, and resource constraints might not allow the team to complete all steps in the ideal way. Project management tools can help teams ensure that all steps are appropriately addressed, however.

If team members have external pressure and workload imposed upon them, the team leader should be flexible and look for ways to decrease the complexity of the project. Breaking the steps of the PET process down into manageable portions can help to decrease complexity. For example, in planning to translate findings from an EBP project that entail implementing a new system for monitoring intracranial pressure, team members might need to "divide and conquer." They could divide up sections of the protocol and current self-learning packet to be revised as part of this change. The astute team leader can help re-allocate tasks, as needed.

Artful planning is at its best when the team tries to predict where barriers or risks might occur in the process and determines ways to manage these risks. The EBP team should always ask the question, "What can go wrong?", when developing the project plan. Some problems can be predicted, for example, if the translation plan includes procurement of new equipment, the risk exists that the equipment will not be available at the time it is needed. Other risks are harder to foresee, for example, the pilot unit has staffing problems because of a flu outbreak and cannot execute the planned change in the requested time frame. The project plan should allocate time to account for unanticipated problems or should include developed contingency plans.

Establishing Controls

Establishing controls allows for successful completion of an EBP project. Examples include establishing milestones, monitoring the project plan, tracking costs, and defining a communication plan.

Milestones are useful to help the team to monitor its progress. Clear, unambiguous milestones, or targets, describe what is to be done within a stated time frame. For example, during the evidence phase of PET, one milestone might be to conduct an internal and external search for evidence by May 2009; another milestone might be to complete appraisal of all evidence collected by June 2009. Setting milestones is often based on the WBS or the Gantt chart. Milestones allow team members to have shared goals, and charts provide a visual mechanism for tracking progress.

The team should track and review the project on a regular basis and identify any areas in which changes to the plan are required. Monitoring of the project plan helps with early identification of problems with the intended timeline. Tracking milestones enables the team to determine if scheduled tasks have been completed on time. Sometimes the amount of time needed to complete a particular step is underestimated. The extra time required for the nurse to perform the step has an impact on the amount of money charged as indirect time to the unit's budget, so teams want to recognize delays and take corrective action as early as possible.

Tracking costs is another way of establishing controls. Not all EBP projects require additional funding or a formal budget. However, in the spirit of fiscal accountability, the team should still keep track of costs related to the project. For example, a team might incur unanticipated copying and printing costs with respect to the EBP project communication plan. Monitoring such costs calls attention to these expenditures so the team can implement corrective measures, such as a paper-lite strategy. When implementation of a translation strategy requires funding, the team can benefit from a budget. Soliciting the help of departmental administrators or managers who have experience in budget preparation can help a team in anticipating changes that might occur, especially with translation projects that take longer than is expected. After a budget has been developed, the team needs to make certain that costs are controlled as the translation plan is implemented.

Finally, establishing a communication plan serves as another mechanism for keeping the team on course. Having a written communication strategy reminds the team to keep stakeholders informed of progress. This progress reporting generally serves as an incentive to stay on track because delays are noticeable and stakeholders may request corrective action plans.

EBP Project Management Skills and Competencies

EBP is a team effort. Diverse perspectives and experiences add substance to the decision-making process of how to translate findings. Team leaders should assist members of their teams to work interdependently with each other and with project stakeholders. Building an effective EBP team is an ongoing process; the leader plays a key role in helping team members develop competencies required to work effectively in the team. Health care teamwork training competencies have been identified and fall within five competency domains:

- Communication

- Task management

- Situational awareness

- Decision making

- Leadership

   (Clay-Williams & Braithwaite, 2009).

Communication

One of the largest contributors to the success or failure of any project is communication. EBP teams are formed with a mutual purpose. Communication among team members begin with mutual respect for each other and for the skills and knowledge each person brings to the table. Active listening is a prerequisite for communication and includes the actions listed below:

- Pay undivided attention to the speaker

- Refrain from side conversations in group settings

- Use body language to illustrate attention to the speaker's words

- Provide feedback to show understanding about what is said

- Allow the speaker to finish his or her thoughts before offering a response

- Respond appropriately in a candid, respectful manner

Communication can also be enhanced by team members' learning to ask questions to clarify understanding, focus the conversation, discover the speaker's perspective, and challenge the speaker to look at things in a different way. EBP team members should provide timely feedback when requested, using a direct and supportive communication style, and respond in an open and accepting manner when feedback is offered.

Nurses on EBP project teams need to be aware of the communication styles of team members and any cultural or personality factors that have the potential to serve as barriers to effective communication. Leaders of EBP projects should identify appropriate communication channels and should be attentive to the communication needs and styles of team members. Communication should be focused on the goals of the project and ensure that team members receive information needed in a timely manner.

Task Management

The EBP team needs to manage tasks efficiently and effectively. Team members need to manage changing priorities and prioritize critical tasks when necessary. They need to allocate sufficient resources and time to complete tasks, distribute and assign tasks thoughtfully, and re-allocate tasks where required (Clay-Williams & Braithwaite, 2009).

Situational Awareness

Teams require a shared mental model to function. Each team member should understand his or her role, responsibilities, and contribution to the project. Nurses on EBP teams need to be tuned into local unit, departmental, and organizational politics and power structure. Project outcomes that recommend actions contrary to the organization's mission or the agency's policies are doomed to fail. Individual cultural differences and organizational cultural norms influence the buy-in for change, so team members must be aware of how to manage cultural diversity (PMI, 2008).The ability to influence project outcomes requires an understanding of the motivations and concerns of stakeholders, active listening skills, artful negotiation, appreciation for the contributions of others, and expertise in providing and receiving feedback in a constructive manner.

Decision Making

Decision making is critical in the translation stage of the EBP process. After evidence has been compiled, analyzed, and synthesized, the team needs to decide on the translation strategy. Nurse members of EBP teams should understand how to rate the pros and cons of alternatives, select the best solution, secure buy-in for the planned change, plan a pilot, and evaluate achievement of project goals. Mastery of these competencies by all team members ensures that decisions are made through consensus.

Leadership

EBP team leaders should display effective teamwork skills. True leaders can focus the efforts of a group of individuals toward a mutual goal. Trust and respect are critical to this ability. EBP project leaders establish and maintain the vision, keep the team's focus on answering the practice question, discuss opportunities for change, and develop action plans for translation of findings. EBP project leaders should consider the capabilities of other team members to perform assigned tasks. They might be called to back up other team members when the situation warrants. To keep the team engaged, leaders should maintain a positive, supportive attitude and a participative leadership style.

Case in Point

Distractions and Interruptions to Medication Administration

Pediatric nurses at an urban academic medical center wondered if and how distractions and interruptions affect the nurses' ability to complete the five medication rights during medication administration. Looking for clues, the group queried its online event reporting system and conducted staff nurse focus groups. A common theme surfaced; distractions and interruptions were perceived as contributing to lack of completion of the five medication rights.

Armed with this information, the group committed to conducting an EBP project aimed at examining and reducing distractions and interruptions during medication administration. With medication safety as an organizational priority, the nurses focused on ways to manage resource, time, scope, and financial constraints of EBP project implementation.

Overcoming Project Constraints

Resources were needed to complete the project. A team was assembled that consisted of members with combined knowledge, skills, and experience in EBP and project management. The medication safety nurse, a student in a Doctor of Nursing Practice (DNP) program, served as project leader for the pediatric team, which included a nurse manager and a unit-based staff nurse champion. If all members were to contribute fully to the project, everyone needed to have the same basic knowledge about the organizational EBP model.

In a synergistic effort, the team joined forces with the hospital's Nursing Clinical Quality Improvement (NCQI) Committee, whose members were educated in use of the model and served as mentors in EBP project planning and implementation. Mentoring, coupled with easy-to-use tools and written summaries of the project and its relevance to clinical care, helped to develop competence in EBP project management. Further expertise was offered by DNP faculty as the team refined the problem, appraised the evidence, and planned translation strategies. One strategy included an observation of actual interruptions that occurred during medication administration. The project leader garnered additional resources by enlisting the support of students from a school of nursing. This strategy gained the team the support they required and provided students with exposure to and practical experience in the execution of the EBP process.

Allocation of *time* from routine activities to work on the project was a concrete measure of the priority given to this project by nurse leaders who recognized the project's importance to the entire organization. For one year, an hour of each monthly NCQI meeting was devoted to the conduct of the project. Support at the unit-level came from the nurse manager who allocated approximately 20 hours of time, free of patient care duties, to the staff champion to participate in project-related activities. The project leader incorporated the pilot of the evidence-based translation strategies into her DNP coursework. From the beginning, the leader needed to understand, articulate, and mesh expectations from the hospital with the academic program to create a timeline that enabled the two entities to be in sync with each other.

Despite having a well-thought-out and endorsed timeline, things can go awry. To keep the project on track, teams need to anticipate potential stumbling blocks. For example, the team planned to collect baseline data until 304 distractions and interruptions were observed (n=304). They reached the desired sample size quickly after just two days (a Tuesday and a Thursday). The team felt that a reasonable critique would be that they had little variability in data collection days, and they wondered whether more data should be collected on different days. Team members wrestled with issues related to maintaining a quality study, extending the timeline, and re-enlisting the same data collectors. After weighing the short-term impact of additional data collection on the timeline against the long-term impact on study quality, the team decided to collect more data on other days of the week.

The team defined and managed the *scope* of the project for implementation in a single pediatric unit. Discussion of the problem statement and evidence appraisal with NCQI members from other departments enticed the team to consider a variety of avenues to explore. Through an iterative process of refining the problem and critical appraisal of the evidence, the team developed four project aims to guide decisions and maintain the focus on evidence translation:

1. Describe perceived and observed distractions and interruptions during medication administration on a 24-bed adolescent medical-surgical inpatient unit.

2. Examine the relationship between the frequency of observed distractions and interruptions and nurse perceptions of the frequency of distractions and interruptions.

3. Determine if medication storage location influences the frequency and types of distractions and interruptions.

4. Describe the effectiveness of changes within the nurses' work environment, including the education intervention, on actual and perceived distractions and interruptions.

Before selecting a translation strategy, the project leader developed a *budget* to identify associated costs. Although costs were modest, the educational programs developed for this project could not happen without funding. The team proceeded with planning the educational intervention as they investigated funding options. With the encouragement of their mentors, team members applied for and received an award given annually to a nurse-led team proposing the most promising quality improvement/research project focused on patient safety.

Lessons Learned

Here are pearls of wisdom to share about the implementation of an EBP project:

1. **Assemble the right team.** A team can design the perfect project, incorporate the most recent evidence, and develop the most proactive timeline ever, but if it does not have talented and dedicated champions at various leadership and clinical levels, ensuring the project's success is difficult.

2.   **Manage time and timelines efficiently and flexibly.** Clearly articulate the problem, its impact on clinical care, and required resources. Provide a clear action plan to key project stakeholders with milestones and time frames for completion. Maintain a focus on quality. Make adjustments when it can improve the outcome.

3.   **Keep the project focused and sharp.** Create and refer often to the project's "charter," for example, a written summary of the projects aims, objectives, and outcome. This document serves as the project compass. Remain alert for situations that might compromise the scope, intent, and overall success of the project.

4.   **Ask for help and explore all possible sources of funding, when needed.** Don't be bashful! Prepare a list of organizational leaders who might help with funding. Make the business case and sell the idea to each leader on that list. Align the request with the organization's mission, values, or a department's objectives. Answer the question: "What's in it for team members or the organization as a whole?"

5.   **Be passionate and positive.** Select an area of practice change that intrigues and motivates the team. Enthusiasm (or lack of it) can transfer to others, so maintain genuine eagerness even when things don't go as planned. "Successful thinking" leads to a successful EBP project.

Conclusion

Successful projects meet their scope, time, resource, and cost goals. Team members feel a sense of accomplishment when the well-planned project enables them to answer the practice question, develop and implement translation strategies, and evaluate the impact of the change strategy and progress to desired outcomes. By effectively managing EBP projects, nurses experience a high degree of satisfaction in knowing that the best available evidence has been translated into practice. Project management knowledge and skills allow nurses to gain confidence in their ability to seek out, appraise, and translate evidence into practice. With each new EBP project, the nurse gains expertise to assist colleagues in answering future EBP questions.

References

Association for Project Management. (2006). *APM Body of Knowledge definitions* (5th ed.). Bedfordshire, UK: APM Publishing.

Clay-Williams, R. & Braithwaite, J. (2009). Determination of health-care teamwork training competencies: A Delphi study. *International Journal for Quality in Health Care 21,* (6), pp. 433–440.

Gantt, H. L. (1974). *Work, wages, and profits.* Easton, Pennsylvania: Hive Publishing Company.

Ginn, D. & Varner, E. (2004). The design for Six Sigma Memory Jogger: Tools and methods for robust processes and products. Salem, NH: Goal/QPC.

Internet Center for Management and Business Administration, Inc. (2007). PERT. Retrieved June 29, 2009, from www.netmba.com/operations/project/pert

Kaufman, D. S. (2005). Using project management methodology to plan and track inpatient care. *Joint Commission Journal on Quality and Patient Safety, 31*(8), pp. 463–468.

Lipshutz, A.K.M., Fee, C., Schell, H., Campbell, L., Taylor, J., Sharpe, B. A., Nguyen, J., & Gropper, M.A. (2008). Strategies for success: A PDSA analysis of three QI initiatives in critical care. *The Joint Commission Journal on Quality and Patient Safety, 34*(8), pp. 435–444.

Newhouse, R. P., Dearholt, S. L., Poe, S. S., Pugh, L. C., & White, K. M. (2007). *Johns Hopkins Nursing Evidence-based practice model and guidelines.* Indianapolis, IN: Sigma Theta Tau International.

Pearce, C. (2007). Ten steps to carrying out a SWOT analysis. *Nursing Management UK, 14*(2), p. 25.

Project Management Institute, Inc. (2008). *A guide to the Project Management Body of Knowledge. (PMBOK guide).* (4th ed.). Newtown Square, Pennsylvania: Project Management Institute, Inc.

Schwalbe, K. (2007). *Information technology project management* (5th ed.). Boston, MA: Thomson Course Technology.

7

Measuring and Managing EBP Outcomes

The most important mandate in today's health care environment is preserving and enhancing quality of care while delivering services in the most efficient and cost effective manner (Schuster, McGlynn and Brook, 2005). One response to this mandate certainly has been the creation of programs to measure and manage outcomes of care. The goal of having an evidence-based practice (EBP) is to assure the highest quality of care by using evidence to promote optimal outcomes.

A major current health care political debate centers around the use of comparative effectiveness research (CER), which is the generation and synthesis of evidence that compares the benefits and harms of alternative methods to prevent, diagnose, treat, and monitor a clinical condition or to improve outcomes and the delivery of care. The purpose of CER is to assist consumers, clinicians, purchasers, and policy makers in making informed decisions to improve outcomes of health care at both the individual and population levels, and CER is viewed as a viable way to help drive down spiraling health care costs while continuing to provide quality care (Institute of Medicine, 2009).

Block (2006) has identified factors that have created the demand for outcomes measurement and management:

1. Need to define quality (and quantify that definition)

2. Need to measure effectiveness and appropriateness of care

3. Need to contain costs in health care (efficiency)

4. Outcry for safety in health care

5. Demand by providers in EBP environment to choose appropriate and effective care and treatments

6. Demand by purchasers for value (balance of cost and effectiveness)

7. Demand by consumers for information and transparency about health care

8. Tremendous variability in health care

9. Need to provide benchmarks

10. Need to report and compare

What Are Outcomes?

We usually think of outcomes in our practices as a measurable change in the health status or behavior of the client. Health care providers have been measuring outcomes for over 150 years. Florence Nightingale measured and wrote about outcomes of care during the Crimean War in the mid-1800s. In 1917, a physician named Ernest Codman called for the implementation of a program that he referred to as the end-result idea. He called on hospitals to measure and make public the "end results" of patient care to improve the practice of their staff. He was labeled an eccentric by his peers, and we really didn't hear much more about outcomes for another 50 years. But in the epilogue of his 1917 End Result Hospital report, he says, "Who knows but someday a copy of this book may be dusted off in a library and shown to some lonely hospital trustee. I'm convinced that if a single great general hospital did this thoroughly that other hospitals will have to follow" (Codman, 1917). We are now all following his dream.

Framework for Evaluation

Modern outcomes evaluation in health care began with the work of Avedis Donabedian (1966) who discussed a framework for evaluation of quality care that included three dimensions:

1. Structure—What is the physical location where care is provided, the philosophy of care, or such things as staffing ratios, availability or type of facilities and/or equipment?

2. Process of care—What is being done? Was appropriate treatment provided? Was it done correctly?

3. Outcomes of care—What are the results of the actions?

This framework is still important in health care evaluation today. However, when relating the framework of quality to health care, we have seen a shift in focus over time from structures (having the right things in place) to processes (doing the right things) to most recently an emphasis on outcomes (having the right things happen).

Types of Outcomes

In the nursing literature, some have proposed different classifications or schemas for outcomes evaluation. Lang and Marek (1990) listed 15 measures of effectiveness in nursing: physiological, psychosocial, functional, behavior, knowledge, symptom control, home maintenance, well-being, goal attainment, patient satisfaction, safety, nursing diagnosis resolution, frequency of services, cost of care, and rehospitalization. Lohr (1988) discussed the five Ds of negative outcomes: death, disease, disability, discomfort, and dissatisfaction. Hegyvary (1991) proposed four categories of outcomes assessment: clinical, functional, financial, and perceptual. Jennings, Staggers, and Brosch (1999), while reviewing the literature, discussed three categories of outcomes indicators that they found: patient-focused, provider-focused, and organization-focused outcomes. They mentioned a fourth category, population-focused outcomes, but did not discuss it.

From years of work and research in cost and outcomes of care, this author describes five types of outcomes important to both direct and indirect nursing practice:

- Clinical

- Functional

- Perceptual

- Process or intervention

- Utilization or administrative

When translating evidence into practice, nurses need to use a specific and comprehensive outcomes framework that allows consideration for measurement of all outcome categories that might be important (Kleinpell, 2001, Flarey, 1997).

Clinical Outcomes

Clinical outcomes are patient-focused or disease-specific. These are the outcomes with which we are most familiar; they are physiologic indicators and are more typically focused on a certain aspect of an illness. For example, clinical outcomes measure changes in vital signs, laboratory values, weight gain or loss, or wound healing.

Functional Outcomes

Functional outcomes measure patients' responses and their adaptation to health problems, including maintenance of or improvement in their physical functioning and how well they are living with their particular problem. Examples of functional outcomes include the patient's ability to perform activities of daily living (ADLs) and independent activities of daily living (IADLs) such as being able to shop for food, go to church or synagogue, visit the physician's office, and have their prescriptions refilled. Functional outcomes also include the measurement of quality of life. Typical measurement tools such as the SF12 or SF36 assess how well the patient feels he is coping, how he feels about living with his disease, and whether or not the disease is interfering with his quality of life.

Perceptual Outcomes

Perceptual outcomes focus on a patient's self-report of her experience with care, her satisfaction with care that has been given to her, how well she feels she related with her providers, and her report of or demonstration of knowledge about her disease or treatment regimen. Patient education is inherent in many nursing interventions and an essential measure of nursing care. Perceptual outcomes also include provider satisfaction with care and the work environment.

These outcomes have become increasingly important in nursing and health care. When implementing any type of evidence into practice, organizations must consider the satisfaction of both patients and nurses.

Process or Intervention Outcomes

Process or intervention outcomes measure the appropriateness of treatment or care, that is, what the provider orders or does that affects all of the other outcome measures. Process measures are provider-focused. In the evaluation of implementing evidence into practice, much of what we measure in health care today concerns these process or intervention measures. For example, most of The Joint Commission core measures are process or intervention measures and were developed to increase the likelihood that strong research findings would be implemented into everyday clinical practice. Evidence-based, nursing-specific process measures used in everyday practice include implementation of fall precautions, turning schedules to prevent pressure ulcers, and medication reconciliation to prevent medication errors.

Utilization or Administrative Outcomes

Utilization or administrative outcomes are organization-focused and generally measure the quality of care by the institution or facility as a whole. Usually quantitative, these measures are typically aggregated across patients to provide evidence of an organization's effectiveness. Some of these measures, such as morbidity and mortality rates, have been around for a long time, but administrative outcomes also include measures such as length of stay, cost of care (total and specific types of care such as laboratory costs, pharmacy costs, and so on), number of emergency department visits, admission rates, and readmission rates.

Outcomes Evaluation

Outcomes evaluation includes both measurement and management of outcomes.

- Outcomes measurement deals with describing and/or quantifying outcomes.

- Outcomes management is the process designed to provide safe, timely, effective, efficient, equitable, patient-centered, quality, and accessible health care.

Thus, outcomes evaluation is at the heart of all EBP work. It is the bottom line of any evidence implementation and looks at the impact of the evidence on cost, quality, performance, and productivity. How do you decide what to measure, and after you have decided, how are you going to measure in the phenomenon of interest? Most importantly, you have to answer this question: What happens to a patient as a result of implementing this evidence into practice? Have you been able to improve, or at least maintain, outcomes of care while implementing this new evidence into practice?

Outcomes evaluation usually serves two purposes: quality improvement internally to improve practice and accountability externally to decrease practice variations and to compare practice to benchmarks and make improvements. Organizations meet both of these purposes when evaluating outcomes of implementing evidence into practice.

According to McGlynn (1996), the purposes of outcomes measurement are as follows:

1. Provide information for consumer choice for health care providers or for treatment choices

2. Design financial incentives to achieve cost containment, access, or quality of care

3. Identify areas in which quality should be improved

4. Monitor and evaluate changes in policy or new treatments

President Clinton's Advisory Commission on Consumer Protection and Quality in the Health Care Industry through a Strategic Framework Board did a lot of work on identifying a common set of quality measures for the nation (these measures can be found at http://www.hcqualitycommission.gov/final/). One of the most interesting aspects of the work of this Strategic Framework Board was the development of guiding principles for selection of measures (McGlynn, 2003):

1. The measure should link directly to a national goal.

2. The intended use of the measure should be clear and compelling.

3. The common set should be parsimonious.

4. The common set should not impose undue burden on those who provide data.

5. The common set should help providers improve the delivery of care.

6. The common set should help all stakeholders make more informed decisions.

7. The common set should be improved over time based on feedback from providers and other key users of the information.

The objectives of parsimony and avoiding undue burden imply that the common set of measures is a small number of key measures that are useful for both choice and improvement rather than a comprehensive set of all acceptable measures.

This national work has direct application to any nursing practice, and the guiding principles are important factors to consider when deciding what to measure to evaluate the effectiveness of implementing evidence into practice.

Selecting the outcomes to be measured in your practice is both important and challenging. Planning is critical to the success of an outcomes measurement project. In identifying the outcomes, those involved need to understand what is to be measured, why the measurement is critical to patient care (internal and/or external reasons), and the impact of the outcomes measurement plan. Mapping the process for all who are involved in the data collection can be helpful. The development or adoption of a specific data-gathering tool to collect outcomes data can assist the process and ensure that the outcomes are collected and documented in a consistent manner. Give consideration to these issues when choosing or developing an outcomes measurement tool or instrument:

- Patient population

- Setting

- Purpose of measurement

- Outcomes definition

- Measurement specifications

- Timing (when to be collected and for how long)

Outcomes Evaluation Process

The process of outcomes measurement and management involves seven distinct steps:

1. Problem description

2. Outcome description

3. Team building

4. Outcome measurement plan

5. Data collection

6. Data analysis and presentation

7. Translation of evidence into practice

Problem Description

Identify the area of weakness that you have on your unit and prioritize the focus on something about which your organization cares, such as a high cost, high volume, or high risk problem, to get the resources (time, people, and money) for the project. Determine the focus of implementing the evidence into practice: performance improvement, safety initiative, pilot study, or research. Finally, ask yourself who wants the information, what do they want to know, and why do they want to know it, so you can figure out who is really interested in this and design the outcomes evaluation process appropriately.

Outcome Description

The second step in the outcomes evaluation process is to identify, define, and describe the outcomes to be measured. At this step in the process most nurses look for assistance and search for appropriate outcomes to measure. First, decide what is important to measure about this evidence implementation. Are there only clinical concerns or are there also perceptual and administrative outcomes? For example, if you were going to compare the effectiveness of using multidose inhalers compared to nebulizers for treating pediatric patients receiving beta-agonist therapy in the emergency room for an acute exacerbation of asthma, you would be concerned not only about improvement in arterial blood gases and the effect of the medication on heart rate, but also about the time spent in the emergency department and the rate of hospital admission. Think about all five types of outcomes to be sure that you have considered all areas important to your evidence implementation. Remember to keep it as simple as possible and the number of outcomes to be collected to five or less.

You might also look at best practice organizations, places which you might have read or that you heard are doing something in a particular area of interest to help you select the outcome measures for your evaluation. Benchmarking is another strategy to help identify outcomes measures. Look for measures that are being collected by an organization that is similar to your organization or those organizations known as centers for excellence in the clinical area. These organizations might also have a clinical practice guideline for care with specific outcome measures.

Also, state and national sources of outcomes measures—the National Database of Nursing Quality Indicators (NDNQI), Quality Indicator Project, the Institute for Healthcare Improvement (IHI), National Guidelines Clearinghouse (NGC), and the Agency for Healthcare Research and Quality (AHRQ)—can easily be accessed through the Internet. Last, many nursing specialty organizations and the American Nurses Association (ANA) have developed standards of practice or clinical practice guidelines that might also be useful. For any specific clinical problem, you can find many examples of outcome measures applicable to your situation. Your organization need not struggle to develop outcomes measures if this is not your strength, and using published outcome measures that can be benchmarked against other organizations has advantages.

Team Building

The next step in the outcomes evaluation process is to build your team. Interestingly, this outcomes evaluation process parallels the Practice question, Evidence, and Translation (PET) process and uses the same principles for developing good teams and positive multidisciplinary collaborations. In health care today, anytime you have a problem in the clinical area and need to collect data, consider who needs to be involved in the particular process. Develop agreement on the problem, what outcomes need to be measured, and what data need to be collected. Discuss which professionals might have an impact on the process, might help with the data collection, or might be a barrier to collecting the data in which you are interested. Involve those stakeholders in defining the problem even if it means beginning your process over again. Identify the experts, facilitators, and champions and determine what expertise you need for the implementation. Consider whether or not all of these individuals need to be involved in the whole process. If you have a culture of inclusiveness, everyone involved in the clinical issue during the implementation might have to be a member of the team. Be aware of the need for buy-in and collaboration. Politically, collaboration can buy a lot of support in the process.

Finally, be cautious in the outcomes evaluation process as the team develops and makes decisions. Every time a decision is made in the process, be disciplined to write the decisions down either in meeting minutes or the project plan. This record keeping is important for standardization and replication purposes and for responding to questions from a late-to-the-table expert who might wonder why you did or did not do something. For example, you might have a record that the seven of those involved in the second meeting of the team discussed and made a decision to exclude or not to exclude a certain group of patients in the evaluation. This documentation can also help you during the analysis, recommendations, and translation phase of the project as it serves as a record of decisions made during team meetings.

Outcome Measurement Plan

The next phase of the outcomes evaluation process is to determine how the outcomes are going to be measured for this project. To properly measure identified outcomes, determine the type of data needed and available to measure the chosen outcomes. For example, if you are interested in measuring the cost of care, you would need administrative data that might come from a hospital finance database, insurance claims, or a laboratory or pharmacy system. Clinical data are usually available from patient records.

Next, discuss with the team how much data is needed (number of cases, charts, months, and so on) and how long the data is going to be collected. The length of time for data collection is determined by the number of cases you need to show a difference. In quality improvement, the length of time might be short if you are using a rapid cycle model of improvement. However, you might need several months of data collection if you are looking at a particular patient flow issue or a satisfaction issue to ensure that you can see if a change occurred.

Then, determine who is going to collect the data, which involves knowing if the data collection is to be original data generation to inform this particular project or data coming from reports supplied to your team. Always look for the simplest source and route to obtain required data. Unfortunately, nurses are often identified as the easiest way to obtain data. However, before you ask the nurses to collect the data, be certain that no one else is already collecting the outcomes of interest.

Finally, consider if anything might relate to or influence the outcome measure, such as risk factors or variables that might confound the outcomes you are measuring. If you find any factors, consider how you can measure or control that influence on your outcome. For example, you discovered research evidence from the literature that a particular intervention for congestive heart failure patients (high cost and high volume problem) improved outcomes and decreased hospital readmission rates. What factors might confound measuring outcomes in heart failure patients? Consider how different insurance companies handle the management of heart failure patients. Consider age and co-morbid condition differences in these patients. After you have identified those things that might affect outcomes evaluation, then determine how you might try to control for or at least measure and account for these differences. In this example, you might consider including type of insurance, age, and other co-morbidities as data or variables that you collect.

Data Collection

The decision about how and where to record the data is usually one of the hardest to make. Evaluate the availability of an electronic infrastructure within your organization to determine if the data has to be collected manually or if it can be made available through some type of information technology platform, such as a handheld device or use of a data collection tool that can be scanned directly into a database.

At this stage of the process, you need to monitor and evaluate the accuracy and integrity of the data you are collecting. Did you encounter any important barriers to data access that you had not foreseen and included in your plan? Were the data available and collected according to plan? Consider the reliability of the data collection process and if the results you collected were consistent and replicable. For example, if you measured the same variable in the same way again, would you get the same result? Finally, determine the validity of the measurement technique you are using. In other words, is the data being collected measuring what it is supposed to measure?

Data Analysis and Presentation

After data collection is complete, analyze and present the results of the data collection. You might need a statistician on the outcomes evaluation team to assist you to pick the appropriate statistical tests to analyze the data.

Case in Point

Statistical Concepts Related to Outcomes Evaluation

Key statistical concepts include levels of measurement, measures of central tendency, measures of variability/dispersion, measures related to tools/instruments, and statistical tests used in outcomes evaluation.

Levels of Measurement

1. Nominal data: Frequency, count, or categories of data with no rankings. This is the lowest level of measurement because nominal data represent only the categories or classifications and do not have a numerical value attached to it that would make one category better than another. Examples of nominal data include gender, marital status, educational level, type of insurance, or yes/no answers to questions (for example, "Does your patient have diabetes mellitus?").

2. Ordinal data: Also categories of data, but these data have some rank based upon the relative amounts of the characteristic of the data of interest. However, no measurable quantitative differences or equality can be measured in the ranks. Likert scales are often used when measuring ordinal data with categories such as strongly agree, agree, neutral, disagree, and strongly disagree. Familiar examples of ordinal data are patient satisfaction scores that use a similar scale.

3. Interval data: Data where the differences between the measurements have meaning and show rankings on a scale with equal intervals. However, in interval data the zero point is arbitrary. An example of interval data is temperature.

4. Ratio data: Data variables on scales that have equal intervals and an absolute zero point. This is the highest level of measurement. Examples of ratio data include age, intake and output, weight, pulse, and length of stay

Measures of Central Tendency

- Mean: The average

- Median: The middle

- Mode: The most frequent

Measures of Variability/Dispersion

- Range: The range of values

- Normal distribution: Distributed data has something like a "bell curve" shape.

- Standard deviation: A statistic that tells you how tightly all the various examples are clustered around the mean in a set of data. When the examples are tightly bunched together and the bell-shaped curve is steep, you have a small standard deviation. When the examples are spread apart and the bell curve is relatively flat, you have a relatively large standard deviation.

Measures Related to Tools/Instruments

- Reliability: The consistency with which an instrument measures the outcome and accurately reflects the true measure of the attribute.

- Validity: Three important types in outcomes measurement.

  - Content: Does the instrument adequately cover the content area?

  - Criterion: Is there a relationship between scores on the instrument and some external criterion?

  - Construct: What construct is the instrument actually measuring?

Simple Statistical Tests Used in Outcomes Evaluation

- Chi square analysis: Comparison of categories of data

- T-Tests: Comparison of means

- Pearson's r: Correlation or relationship between variables

The entire multidisciplinary team should be involved in the analysis of findings and the discussion of results for a complete interpretation and to make the most information out of the data for dissemination of the results. The team should decide who is going to receive the results, what type of report format to use, and if the team is going to do a written report, a verbal presentation, or both. As the findings are presented, involve the staff in discussion about their interpretation of the findings or lack of findings. They are often the best analyzers in the process and might have additional insight into the findings.

Translation of Evidence into Practice

The last step in the outcomes evaluation process is to apply the findings to the practice question. Again, the team must be involved in the decision making and agree about any type of practice change or resource allocation to implement from the evaluation. You also need a plan for follow-up evaluation for any change made. The team also has an obligation to disseminate the findings to other health care professionals both in your facility and outside so that others can learn from your experience.

Case in Point

Using the Outcomes Evaluation Process to Address Patient Falls

As an example to put evidence-based interventions into practice to decrease patient falls, follow the seven steps of the outcomes evaluation process.

Describe the Problem

In the typical general medicine unit in a hospital today, with a majority of patients over 65 years of age, falls prevention is a unit priority. Falls have been identified as a nursing-sensitive outcome measure, making this an appropriate concern for an outcomes evaluation process. The practice question is this: What are the evidence-based best practice strategies to decrease fall rates? Begin addressing the question by searching the evidence to develop evidence-based intervention strategies.

Describe the Outcome

What type of data do you need to evaluate your intervention strategies? Consider the five types of outcomes. The most important outcome is fall rates, which is a clinical outcome measure. Where can you collect or obtain this data? Fall rates might come from risk management or from the NDNQI database if your hospital is collecting those data.

What other outcome data is important? If you are putting falls-risk patients on beds with alarms, you might be interested in whether this affects their satisfaction or experience in your facility. Measuring this experience would be a perceptual outcome measure. What if one of the evidence-based strategies suggested using "sitters" for those identified to be at risk? You could hire sitters, or you could involve family members to "sit." How you implement this piece of evidence determines how you evaluate the strategy. However, remember that you need to collect enough data to have a good evaluation, but also want to keep it simple to limit the burden on any data collectors.

Build the Team

Decide who needs to be involved in improving the fall rate on your unit. Consider all the expertise you need to implement the intervention, identify leadership needed to conduct the intervention, include those who might supply or collect the outcome measures, and identify champions from the staff at all levels.

Determine How Outcomes Will Be Measured

How long will you have to collect the outcome measures to see impact of the translation of the intervention? You might need to look at how many falls you have on your unit or in your department per quarter. Also, decide on how you are going to obtain the data or who you might have to ask to collect the data.

You must carefully think through the process and discuss it with your team so you don't leave anything out. Decide how you are going to record the data if you have to collect it. Are you going to have to design a data collection tool or can you record in a current part of the record? Will it be recorded manually or electronically, and how are the measures of interest going to be entered into the database for analysis? Finally, discuss with the team if any confounders or other things might influence your evaluation of the intervention strategy. Those data should also be identified and a decision made as to whether you want to collect or obtain them.

Your evidence search shows that best practice organizations are routinely doing falls risk assessments on every patient on admission and on certain categories of patients regularly during their hospital stay. Collecting and receiving those data can give you information on when falls happen, the patient profile of fallers, and what trends put those patients at risk (medications, diagnoses, age, gender, support of significant others, and so on). Again, remember only to collect enough additional data to inform your evaluation; keep it simple and limit the burden on any data collectors.

Collect the Outcome Data

After these decisions have been made, you can begin data collection recording all agreed upon data points and record them on the form that was developed to collect the data specific to this project. Educate all involved to the data collection process and provide regular updates to the team about the status of the data collection.

Analyze and Present the Results

Were you able to collect the data that you planned? If not, you will have to revise your plan for evaluation. Develop a database using a statistical program so that you are able to run a statistical analysis on the data you collected. The data analysis begins at the identified timeframe for the project. Present the results to the team first for discussion and interpretation. Then, disseminate the results broadly to the organization and beyond if significant findings would help others to improve practice.

Apply the Findings to Practice

After the evaluation is complete, you have to plan to apply the findings to practice and influence the change. Are you going to continue with the intervention as implemented or make changes to it based on the evaluation? You must discuss plans for longer term sustainability of the implementation with the team. Identify the necessary leadership support and additional stakeholders that might have to be involved and determine what resources you need to fully implement and sustain the evidence-based strategies broadly and permanently.

Factors Influencing Outcomes Measurement

Before we finish this chapter, we need to mention other important factors that influence outcomes measurement in health care. The purpose and goal of any outcome measurements must be identified and transparent to all involved in the process. Are the outcomes being collected because of a regulatory or legislative mandate or is the work for internal quality improvement or EBP implementation? Those involved in the outcomes measurement need to understand the end goal of their efforts. To achieve maximum cooperation for data collection, provide routine data reports to those collecting the data for two reasons. First, those involved in the data collection should regularly see what they have collected and how their efforts matter. Second, the data should be provided and discussed regularly to ensure that what is being measured is what was intended and that the outcome is the appropriate measure to be collecting.

You also need to consider the following important challenges when measuring outcomes.

1. Attribution: What part of the outcome measure can be attributed to the provider? What other factors affect the outcomes? What has the most impact on outcomes? Does a cause and effect relationship really exist if that is what you are interested in measuring?

2. Reliability and validity of measures: Whenever possible, use instruments that have been tested and used by others and measures that have been tested and are evidence-based. Take advantage of the many national sources of outcomes measures available. If reliable and valid measures are not available, the team might have to develop measures or a data collection tool specifically for this project. If this latter scenario is the case, then the other challenges discussed in this section become even more important to consider and to remain aware of throughout the project.

3. Aggregation: Many outcome measures are at the patient or individual level. Consider if you can aggregate the measure and still preserve what it is supposed to measure. For example, you might need to decide whether to report your outcome in percentages or raw numbers based on the goal for collecting that outcome.

4. Patient-reported outcomes: These outcomes focusing on well-being, health status, quality of life, patient experience, and patient satisfaction (currently a hotly debated and controversial issue). Much current research examines the reliability and validity of these measures. However, patient-reported measures in the form of surveys and questionnaires are often used because they are more practical and less costly to obtain than observational measures.

Ethical Considerations

Ethical considerations are paramount in any type of outcomes measurement in health care. The ethics of outcomes evaluation requires us to consider the way in which intended users of outcomes data might respond to that data, how they might use the data, and whether or not they are going to use it to improve practice and the delivery of health care. Again, when considering the ethics of outcomes evaluation, you face questions about the source, reliability, and objectivity of the outcomes data, including the validity of any conclusions or inferences drawn from the data to create information. Often when you discuss the use or misuse of outcomes data that might or might not be risk- or case-mix adjusted for direct comparison of the performance of two providers, organizations, or programs, you face an important ethical question. This question arises because when you compare performance, unless outcomes data are risk- or case-mix adjusted, variations among providers or organizations have no meaning.

Additional ethical concerns arise over the release of outcomes data to public reporting and pay-for-performance/quality programs, the provision of incentives to providers, denial of care, and the potential use of those data in malpractice or negligence cases. Finally, you must consider the use of any protected health information, governed by the Health Insurance Portability and Accountability Act (HIPAA), when designing outcomes evaluation. Although an Institutional Review Board (IRB) application is not usually required for internal quality improvement or EBP projects, you can request an IRB opinion about the outcomes data collection to ascertain whether or not the evaluation involves acting for the good of the patient in the use of the data.

Outcomes Measures in Nursing

The role for nursing in outcomes evaluation includes determining what should be measured and defining how outcomes can be positively influenced through nursing care at all levels, including the individual patient level, the unit level, and the organizational/agency/practice level. Traditional outcomes measures such as mortality, morbidity, length of stay, cost, and readmission have not reflected nursing contribution to health care. We now have many more choices for measuring the outcome of nursing care.

National Database for Nursing Quality Indicators

The National Center for Nursing Quality at the American Nurses Association developed a set of nursing sensitive measures that are housed in the National Database of Nursing Quality Indicators (NDNQI), the only database of nursing indicators collected at the unit level (see Table 7.1).

Go to https://www.nursingquality.org/ for more information about the NDNQI.

Table 7.1: Nursing-Sensitive Measures from the National Database of Nursing Quality Indicators

National Database of Nursing Quality Indicators (NDNQI)

Indicator	Sub-indicator	Type of Measure(s)
1. Nursing Hours per Patient Day	a. Registered Nurses (RN) b. Licensed Practical/Vocational Nurses (LPN/LVN) c. Unlicensed Assistive Personnel (UAP)	Structure
2. Patient Falls		Process & Outcome
3. Patient Falls with Injury	a. Injury Level	Process & Outcome
4. Pediatric Pain Assessment, Intervention, Reassessment (AIR) Cycle		Process
5. Pediatric Peripheral Intravenous Infiltration Rate		Outcome

continues

Indicator	Sub-indicator	Type of Measure(s)
6. Pressure Ulcer Prevalence	a. Community Acquired b. Hospital Acquired c. Unit Acquired	Process & Outcome
7. Psychiatric Physical/Sexual Assault Rate		Outcome
8. Restraint Prevalence		Outcome
9. RN Education/Certification		Structure
10. RN Satisfaction Survey Options	a. Job Satisfaction Scales b. Job Satisfaction Scales – Short Form c. Practice Environment Scale (PES)	Process & Outcome
11. Skill Mix: Percent of total nursing hours supplied by	a. RNs b. LPN/LVNs c. UAP d. % of total nursing hours supplied by Agency Staff	Structure
12. Voluntary Nurse Turnover		Structure
13. Nurse Vacancy Rate		Structure
14. Nosocomial Infections (Pending for 2007)	a. Urinary catheter-associated urinary tract infection (UTI) b. Central line catheter-associated blood stream infection (CABSI) c. Ventilator-associated pneumonia (VAP)	Outcome

Reprinted from Montalvo, I., (September 30, 2007)

National Quality Forum

The National Quality Forum (NQF), "a nonprofit organization that aims to improve the quality of health care for all Americans," also has as part of its mission the setting of national priorities and goals for performance improvement and the endorsing national consensus standards for measuring and publicly reporting on performance (NQF, 2009). NQF has endorsed 15 nursing-sensitive outcome measures as part of its Quality Data Set (QDS) and provides a common technological framework for defining clinical data necessary to measure performance and accelerate improvement in patients' quality of care (see Table 7.2).

Table 7.2: National Voluntary Consensus Standards for Nursing-Sensitive Care

---

Performance Measures

1. Death Among Surgical Inpatients with Treatable Serious Complications (Failure to Rescue)

2. Pressure Ulcer Prevalence

3. Patient Falls

4. Falls with Injury

5. Restraint Prevalence (vest and limb)

6. Catheter-Associated Urinary Infection (CAUTI) Rate for Intensive Care Unit (ICU) Patients

7. Central Line-Associated Bloodstream Infection (CLABSI) Rate for Intensive Care Unit (ICU) and Neonatal Intensive Care Unit (NICU) Patients

8. Ventilator-Associated Pneumonia (VAP) Rate for Intensive Care Unit (ICU) and Neonatal Intensive Care (NICU) Patients

9. Smoking Cessation Counseling for Acute Myocardial Infarction (AMI)

10. Smoking Cessation Counseling for Heart Failure (HF)

11. Smoking Cessation Counseling for Pneumonia (PN)

12. Skill Mix

13. Nursing Care Hours per Patient Day

14. Practice Environment Scale-Nursing Work Index (PES-NWI)

15. Voluntary Turnover

(Joint Commission, 2005)

Nursing Care Outcomes

Nurses in all roles, specialties, and settings are interested in an almost endless list of types of outcomes measurement. Here is a list of outcomes worth mentioning that might help you to think about how you could measure improvement in your practice change implementation:

1. Appropriateness of care (adherence to professional standards)— Necessary, overuse, or underuse for impact (high volume, high cost, high risk) diseases: Diabetes mellitus, asthma, hypertension, depression, cardiac disease, mental health disorders

2. Potentially preventable complications (PPCs)

3. Rates and completeness of immunizations

4. Screening (cancer)

5. General preventive care

6. Prenatal care

7. Risk factors

8. Antibiotic use

9. Quality of life

10. Patient satisfaction

11. Nurse satisfaction

12. Length of stay

13. Cost of care (total or specific service/product line costs)

14. Admission rates

15. Re-admission rates

16. Potentially preventable re-admissions

17. Morbidity

18. Mortality

19. Nurse staffing—RN/LPN/NA rates, vacancy rates, turnover rates, intent to leave

20. Knowledge of self-management strategies for chronic diseases

21. Effects of health problems on ability to function in everyday life

22. Experiences with obtaining care

23. Never events

Advanced practice registered nurses (APRNs) often contribute to required outcomes reporting of measures that might or might not represent a relationship with the care they are providing. APRNs have an obligation to identify outcome measures and routinely measure their practice at the individual and practice level.

Conclusion

Outcomes evaluation provides essential information about the results of nursing care and our interventions to improve quality and safety of patient care. The identification and measurement of appropriate outcomes to evaluate interventions to answer practice questions is critical to the EBP process. Nurses must take a leadership role in EBP implementation to change practice. Through evaluation of outcomes of care, nurses can take credit for the difference they are making in patients' lives and the organizations in which they work.

References

Block, D. (2006). *Healthcare outcomes management: Strategies for Planning and evaluation.* Massachusetts: Jones and Bartlett Publishers.

Codman, E. A. (1917). *A study in hospital efficiency.* Reprinted by The Joint Commission on Accreditation of Healthcare Organizations Press, 1 Renaissance Blvd., Oakbrook Terrace, Illinois 60181, 1996.

Donabedian, A. (1966). Evaluating the quality of medical care. *Milbank Quarterly, 44*(3): pp. 166–203.

Flarey, D. L. (1997). Patient care outcomes: A league of their own. *Outcomes Management for Nursing Practice, 1*(1): pp. 36–40.

Hegyvary, S. T. (1991). Issues in outcomes research. *Journal of Nursing Quality Assurance, 5*(2): pp. 1–6.

Institute of Medicine. (2001). *Crossing the quality chasm: A new health system for the 21st century.* Washington, DC: National Academy Press.

Institute of Medicine. (2009). *Initial national priorities for comparative effectiveness research.* Washington, DC: National Academy Press.

Jennings, B. Staggers, N. and Brosch, L. (1999). A classification scheme for outcomes indicators. Image: *Journal of Nursing Scholarship, 31* (4): 381-388.

Joint Commission, The. (2005). *Implementation guide for the NQF endorsed nursing-sensitive care performance measures.* Chicago, Illinois: Joint Commission.

Kleinpell, R. M. (2001). *Outcomes assessment in advanced practice nursing.* New York: Springer Publishing Company, Inc.

Lang, N. M. & Marek, K. D. (1990). The classification of patient outcomes. *Journal of Professional Nursing, 6*(3): pp. 158–63.

Lohr, K. N. (1988). Outcome measurement: Concepts and questions. *Inquiry, 25*(1): pp. 37–50.

McGlynn, E. (1996). Setting the context for measuring patient outcomes. *New Directions for Mental Health Services, 1996* (71): pp. 19-32.

McGlynn, E. (2003). Selecting common measures of quality and system performance. *Medical Care, 41*(1) supplement: pp. I 39–I 47.

Montalvo, I. (2007). The National Database of Nursing Quality Indicators (NDNQI). *OJIN: The Online Journal of Issues in Nursing, 12*(3): Manuscript 2. Retrieved February 20, 2010, from www.nursingworld.org/MainMenuCategories/ANAMarketplace/ANAPeriodicals/OJIN/TableofContents/Volume122007/No3Sept07/NursingQualityIndicators.aspx

National Quality Forum (NQF). (2009). About NQF. Retrieved November 25, 2009, from http://www.qualityforum.org/About_NQF/About_NQF.aspx

Schuster, M. A., McGlynn, E. A., & Brook, R. H. (2005). How good is the quality of health care in the United States. *Milbank Quarterly, 83*(4): pp. 843–95.

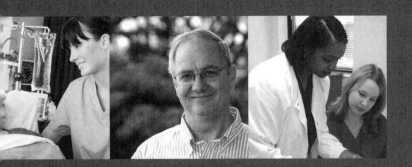

PART III

8

Selecting the Pathway to Translation

The goal of evidence-based practice (EBP) is to "validate current practice or indicate the need to change practice based on evidence" (Newhouse, Dearholt, Poe, Pugh, & White, 2007, p. 37). Modifying or confirming current practice is the ideal product of any EBP project. Whether the decision is to accept evidence-based recommendations to change current practice or to reject these findings and maintain the status quo, the nature and quality of the evidence become the foci of consideration. This chapter explores factors to consider in choosing among alternative options for evidence translation.

Relationship Between Evidence and Translation

Evidence is a function of time. What was the accepted practice guideline yesterday might not be the golden rule today. Clinical practice is dynamic. New technologies and innovations are emerging at a rapid pace. New evidence is continually being generated across settings and has the potential to change prevailing principles and practices.

Developing recommendations for change in systems or processes of care or for maintaining the status quo is the final step in the EBP team's evidence appraisal process, but recommendations alone are not sufficient to affect practice. Final recommendations are the key input into the translation course of action. Translation can take a variety of paths, and the course taken is the result of a complex decision-making process that is linked to a number of factors:

- Consistency or congruence of findings

- Quantity of evidence

- Strength and quality of studies

- Other characteristics for consideration

Consistency and Congruence of Evidence

When translating evidence into practice, the team should not rely solely on recommendations from a single study or the opinion of a single expert to reach a decision. Collective evidence that is congruent assures team members by providing a degree of reliability in the findings. Evidence is *congruent* when findings are in agreement or consistent across evidence sources. Consistency in findings imbues recommendations with greater confidence and makes translation decisions easier. Unfortunately, not all EBP projects yield findings that are in agreement. Sometimes, evidence from an EBP practice question yields conflicting or inconsistent findings. Translation decisions become more challenging under these circumstances.

Quantity of Evidence

The search for evidence is an important step in the EBP process. The quantity of evidence is directly related to the judicious use of search terms and choice of publication databases and other evidence sources. Searching for evidence can be difficult and complicated for a novice. Search terms and concepts might not be obvious; the selection of keywords, which serve as the foundation of an effective search, can be a time-consuming and arduous task for novice members of an EBP team (Timmins & McCabe, 2005). Search results might yield too much or too little information. A successful search should deliver articles directly related to the specific EBP practice question. A medical librarian can help in this step of the process.

Sometimes teams find little evidence related to the practice question of interest in the literature. The team should also search for community standards or position statements published by professional organizations. Specialty or health care organization listservs can help in gathering data about community standards. Position statements are generally published on the websites of professional organizations. Communities of practice have become increasingly popular in the health sector as a mechanism for integrating evidence into practice in a social environment of knowledge sharing and knowledge creation (Li, Grimshaw, Nielsen, Judd, Coyte, & Graham, 2009). Each of these resources can help the team to discover nonresearch evidence related to the question.

Occasionally, despite the team's best efforts to find it, little to no evidence is available. In this case, the team might consider a passive strategy such as "watchful waiting" while opting to make no changes to current practice. If the practice question is of continuing interest, the team might repeat the evidence search periodically to keep abreast of the latest knowledge related to the question. Another option is to seek out and join an established learning collaborative, such as that described by Adams and Titler (2009), to maximize resources and available knowledge in the field of interest.

The team can also choose a more proactive path and develop a research project to generate new knowledge. This path is recommended for EBP teams who have experience in developing small pilot studies or who have access to internal or external resources to assist in the development and conduct of research studies.

Strength and Quality of Evidence

In addition to considering the quantity of evidence related to the particular practice question, the effective EBP team navigates through a variety of levels of evidential strength and quality. The process of evidence appraisal is critical to the success of an EBP project; thus, the team should include someone with the expertise, experience, and knowledge to support and facilitate discussion during, clarify misunderstanding during, and guide the appraisal process. The team can also benefit from a framework to guide the appraisal process, such as the Johns Hopkins Nursing Evidence-Based Practice (JHNEBP) Model. The JHNEBP Model categorizes the strengths of evidence into five levels. Level I represents the highest evidence strength and includes controlled, randomized experimental studies; Level V corresponds with the lowest evidence strength and includes expert opinion and organizational review. The JHNEBP also uses a broadly defined quality rating scale that has three different grades, grade A (high quality) to grade C (low quality).

The final grading of each piece of evidence is one component, the decision to accept or reject recommendations. Though research evidence with a more scientific base and a higher quality rating is weighted heavier in the decision-making process, those making the decisions need to take into consideration a number of other factors, such as the appropriateness and feasibility of implementing the recommended change in the particular setting of interest.

Other Characteristics for Consideration

Other characteristics of the evidence that influence the advisability of implementing recommendations include relevance, clinical significance, and applicability and feasibility.

Relevance

When a team assesses the strength and quality of the evidence, it needs to consider the relevance of the evidence reviewed. A team finds evidence related to many interesting facets of practice during an evidence review. The team needs to ask clarifying questions to keep the focus on the specific area of inquiry. How pertinent is the evidence to the specific question of interest? Is it appropriate for the particular setting, patient population, and/or the individual patient for which the practice question was generated?

Every EBP project should have a clear and explicit question and team members who collectively understand the reason for the EBP project. Though it might be tempting to translate incidental findings into practice, the team should stay focused on the original question.

The team also cannot lose sight of the patient in the process of determining relevance of findings. No matter how strong the evidence, or how high the quality of the evidence, teams must evaluate findings in the context of the patient's priorities and experiences. Failure to take into consideration the individual patient's preferences, internal resources, and personal understanding of well-being can lead to inappropriate application of evidence and poor patient outcomes (Nolan & Bradley, 2008). Germane and targeted interventions that are meaningful to the patient, feasible within the particular practice setting, and with which the patient is motivated to comply, have been found to be critical to effective translation of evidence into practice (Hill, 2009). For family-centered evidence-based practices, an understanding of patient/family values and resources are important determinants in the decision to implement recommended changes (Hidecker, Jones, Imiq, &Villarruel, 2009)

Clinical Significance

EBP teams often focus on the statistical significance of the findings and neglect consideration of the clinical significance. Clinical significance is defined as "a conclusion that an intervention has an effect that is of practical meaning to patients and health care providers" (McGraw-Hill Concise Dictionary of Modern Medicine, 2002) A study can be rated high quality because of its statistical significance; however, the statistical effect (for example, a small change in vital signs that is still within normal limits) might have no clinical significance. In addition, a study can be rated as high quality and statistically significant, but the findings might be impractical or too costly to implement.

Applicability and Feasibility

Other attributes in evidence translation are the applicability and feasibility of the evidence to the practice question. Despite the fact that evidence has first-rate strength, high quality, consistent findings, and statistical and clinical significance, it might be insufficient to answer the practice question. To judge the applicability of evidence, the team assesses the appropriateness and validity of the recommendations for the particular setting and population. To determine feasibility, the team examines the balance between benefit and risks of implementing recommendations, taking into consideration the resources available and the readiness for change. Because applicability and feasibility are central aspects in the translation process, implementing EBP findings that are not feasible can result in resistance to change and failed translation.

Possible Outcomes of the Evidence Phase

The EBP translation process has four common pathways to translation:

1. Evidence might be compelling and supportive of a change in practice.

2. Evidence might be good, with consistent results that support a practice change.

3. The team might find good evidence with conflicting results that might or might not support a practice change.

4. The team might find insufficient or no evidence to support a practice change.

Table 8.1 depicts the common translation pathway for EBP projects. In interpreting the table, assume that recommendations are feasible, applicable, and relevant to the question.

Table 8.1: Translation Pathway for EBP Projects

Evidence

	Compelling	Good, consistent	Good, but conflicting	Insufficient/ absent
Make recommended change?	Yes	Consider pilot of change	No	No
Need for further investigation?	No	Yes, particularly for broad application	Yes, consider periodic review for new evidence or development of research study	Yes, consider periodic review for new evidence or development of research study
Risk-benefit analysis	Benefit clearly outweighs risk	Benefit might outweigh risk	Benefit might or might not outweigh risk	Insufficient information to make determination

Compelling Evidence

An EBP project that yields compelling evidence has more than one study with high levels of strength (Level I, II, III) and quality and consistent and relevant findings. In this instance, the focus of translation activities turns to the assessment of organizational readiness to change. Does the change fit in the organization? Who are the key stakeholders in making the practice change? Is the change feasible, cost effective, and manageable with existing resources? How can the organization be prepared for the change in practice?

Case in Point

Selecting a Sedation Scale

Consider the following practice question: "What is the best sedation assessment tool to use for assessing a patient in an acute care hospital?" In the following example, the team found compelling evidence to support a change in practice: standardization of a sedation assessment tool. The focus of translation is to assess the population of patients requiring sedation assessments in the hospital setting and decide which valid and reliable tool is the best fit for the organization. Evaluating the organizational culture and determining implementation steps to initiate a practice change become the focal points.

Introduction

The use of sedative and analgesic medications to moderately sedate patients for uncomfortable and painful procedures is widely practiced in multiple procedure areas at a large northeastern academic medical center. Mandating policy and establishing standards of care related to procedural sedation is the responsibility of the sedation committee. The original policy had been established in 2001 and was based on regulations from the state board of nursing and the community standard at the time. Procedure areas, perianesthesia care settings, and intensive care units had become comfortable using a level-of-consciousness scale that, though widely used, had not been tested for reliability or validity with any of those patient populations. A commitment to EBP led committee members to question whether the current tool was the best available scale to use for monitoring sedation levels across a variety of settings and age groups.

It is widely recognized that sedation occurs across a continuum including the stages of minimal sedation or anxiolysis, moderate sedation, deep sedation, and general anesthesia. Using a sedation scale that is reliable in establishing when a patient has moved from one stage to another and that can communicate this information succinctly to the care team was a priority in selecting a new sedation scale. In addition, committee members wanted to evaluate tools for simplicity and ease of use; adaptability for use in the intensive care unit (ICU), inpatient units, and procedure areas; validity in both adult and pediatric patient populations; and dissimilarity to the current scale so as to avoid unintended consequences during transition.

The committee set a goal of establishing a new sedation scale that was based on evidence. They wrestled with questions such as "Were there reliable and valid tools available to meet the criteria established by the committee?" and "Could a sedation scale be found that would meet the needs for assessing various types of sedation, including nonprocedural sedation of ICU patients?" The committee chair requested that the institution's nursing EBP fellow be assigned to assist with the evidence search, analysis, and synthesis to expedite the achievement of this goal.

Evidence Recommendation

The EBP fellow presented the results of a comprehensive literature search to the sedation committee. In addition, the fellow surveyed all areas of the institution to determine what scales were currently being used in the various departments. The fellow developed a structured table to allow for easy comparison of the multitude of scales uncovered in the evidence search process, including if the scale was currently in use in the institution; the domain assessed by the scale (for example, delirium, consciousness, agitation, or anxiety); the intended population; the number of scale items; the study author(s); the study population; and the published reliability and validity statistics.

On first review of the evidence table, the committee found it apparent that the primary population in which sedation tools had been validated was adult ICU patients. The sedation committee decided to send out a brief survey to other academic medical centers, requesting that they share which sedation assessment tools were being used and in which clinical area(s) they were being utilized. The survey yielded 10 responses with 70% of respondents reporting use of the Richmond Agitation-Sedation Scale (Ely, Truman, Shintani, Thomason, Wheeler et al., 2003) or the Ramsay Sedation Scale (Ramsay, Savege, Simpson & Goodwin, 1974). Respondents were equally split on use of the selected scale house-wide or solely in ICUs.

Translation

Based on the evidence review, the committee narrowed down its selection process to three scales:

1. Richmond Agitation-Sedation Scale (RASS)

2. Ramsay Sedation Scale

3. State Behavioral Scale (Curley, Harris, Fraser, Johnson & Arnold, 2006)

The State Behavioral Scale (SBS), which was being used in the pediatric ICU at the time of this EBP project, was evaluated for the pediatric population. The pros and cons of each tool were discussed with the sedation committee, whose members included an anesthesiologist, nurse educators, nurse managers, nurse clinicians, and a pharmacist. Committee members represented various types of clinical units, including ICUs, procedure areas, and general inpatient areas. Review and analysis focused on scale reliability and validity information, as well as feasibility and appropriateness for the patient populations within these settings.

The Ramsay Scale was eliminated based on its similarity to the current level of consciousness scale with the numbers inverted. Members of the committee strongly agreed that this similarity would lead to confusion and misunderstandings during the translation stage and that this could present a significant patient safety issue.

The committee selected the RASS scale for house-wide implementation. This decision was largely based on several factors. First, the RASS scale was currently being used in most ICUs as an adjunct to the Confusion Assessment Method (CAM-ICU) and would not require a change in practice for these areas. Second, the scale had documented validity and reliability for the domains of consciousness, agitation, and anxiety. Third, the RASS scale succinctly labeled the stages represented in the continuum levels of sedation, allowing for clear communication of each stage among members of the patient care team. Finally, two other large medical centers had responded to the community survey that they were successfully using the RASS scale hospital-wide.

Good Evidence

Sometimes an EBP project yields good evidence with consistent results, but the evidence is mainly drawn from high quality articles with lower levels of strength (Levels III, IV, and V). This class of evidence suggests the change in practice should be considered because implementing this change might be more beneficial to patients than maintaining the status quo, particularly if no risk or minimal risk to implementing the change exists. Further investigation might be needed for broad application or confirmation in some situations. Consider the example regarding fall injury risk assessment that follows.

Implementing a Practice Change

Patient falls continue to be an important clinical problem in acute care settings. In 2006, falls accounted for 13.9% of unintentional injury in patients 55–64 years old and was the number one reason (45.4%) for unintentional injury in patients greater than 65 years old (CDC, 2009). The practice question investigated was this: "What factors increase the risk of injury when a patient falls?" The team conducted a thorough search for evidence. The topic yielded an overwhelming amount of information, so the team narrowed search terms to specifically look at *fall injury* as opposed to *fall risk assessment*. The evidence primarily comprised nonexperimental studies (Level III). The EBP team discussed the findings and decided that it would be beneficial to develop a fall *injury* risk assessment to complement the fall risk assessment tool as part of the hospital's fall protocol. This decision was based on the evidence that presented a good case for increased risk of fall-related fracture and bleeding injury in certain patient populations. The importance of injury risk assessment was corroborated by the team's experience as part of a multi-institutional collaborative on fall management. Implementing this change, despite the lack of compelling Level I and II evidence, was appropriate because of the potential benefit to individual patients and lack of risk.

Conflicting Evidence

A third potential outcome of an EBP project is the finding of good, yet conflicting evidence to support a change. EBP projects that fall into this category generally do not result in a change in practice. Typically, more evidence is needed to confidently make recommendations.

Case in Point

Medication Safety: To Check or Not to Check?

At a large northeastern academic medical center, various hospital medication clinical standards require certain high-risk intravenous medications to be independently double-checked, although the timing of this safety check is variable. In some instances, the clinical standard requires the double-check to be performed immediately before administration (for example, chemotherapy administration); other clinical standards require the independent double-check to be performed "as soon as possible" after medication initiation and dose change (for example, sedation/vasoactive medication). This variation exists because in some clinical circumstances a medication titration needs to be made immediately as it could pose a patient safety risk if the nurse needed to wait for a second person to perform a double-check. When the anticoagulation committee requested that the timeframe for independent double-check be standardized to "immediately before administration," the nursing standard of care committee (NSOC) decided to examine the evidence behind this practice. The EBP question was this: "Does double-check verification of high-risk medications prior to administration decrease medication errors?"

Evidence Recommendation

Using the Johns Hopkins Nursing EBP (JHNEBP) Model and Guidelines, the NSOC identified, reviewed, and appraised 12 articles. One publication reported on the results of a randomized, controlled trial; four presented details related to descriptive studies; three presented systematic reviews; and four expressed the opinions of experts, clinical practice guidelines, or case studies. The overall strength of the evidence was weak, and the results were inconsistent. Although the practice of performing a medication double-check appears to be widely used and accepted in nursing practice, the NSOC found no solid evidence to support this practice. Opinion-based articles were consistent that double-checking medications is helpful in preventing errors; however, recommendations were not specific in providing evidence on how and why this practice is helpful. Clinical significance was not demonstrated because of the time involved in performing double-checks with little demonstrated benefit.

Most studies focused on a specific medication category such as chemotherapy agents, intravenous medication, or blood transfusion. The sample population varied from rehabilitation patients to nursing students, and the studies had no universal definition of medication error. The number of variants made it difficult to summarize the results and make conclusions. The NSOC found little evidence on how to best perform an independent double-check procedure in any of the articles reviewed.

Translation and Lesson Learned

Given conflicting findings, the EBP team faced a dilemma. Should the hospital discontinue all medication double-checks because of the lack of compelling evidence? Should the hospital add additional medications to the list of those for which double-checks are required despite the lack of evidence to do so?

Because of the low level of evidence, the NSOC decided to continue the current practice of double-checking particular medications as outlined by current hospital clinical standards in the absence of evidence that definitely refuted the value of double-checks. These drugs were limited to those identified by the Institute for Safe Medication Practice (2009) as recommended for double-check verification. The group also chose not to add any additional medications that require double-check verification because the benefit of this practice was not substantiated by the literature. In addition, the NSOC decided that a procedure for "How to do medication double-check verification" was needed because the current process was not specified and variation in practice existed across the clinical units. Finally, the NSOC agreed that an investigation of potential technologic solutions, such as bar-coded medication administration, should be explored to determine if double-check verification should be required if medications are prepared and handled correctly each time a dose is administered.

The EBP team concluded not enough evidence existed to change the current practice of "double-checking specific IV medication as soon as possible after initiation" to "double-checking these IV medications prior to administration". Making this change posed barriers to ICUs where it is essential to start medications quickly and titrate rapidly and a second nurse may not be immediately available to double-check the medication thereby delaying therapy and posing more of a patient safety risk. This is particularly true with vasoactive and/or sedating medications used in the ICU setting.

Insufficient Evidence

The last potential outcome category that may be encountered is when findings are insufficient or no evidence is found to either support or refute a change. This class of evidence warrants no change in practice because the evidence is weak and inconsistent or absent. Changing practice would require further investigation or research to confirm recommendations for change. It is important to note that, while the EBP team may be frustrated by finding insufficient evidence related to the practice question, this project outcome is just as important as outcomes in which the team find more compelling evidence.

No Change in Practice

An example of a project where insufficient evidence was found was a project that asked the following practice question: "Does a Lopez valve used at the tip of a nasogastric feeding tube need to be changed every 24 hours?" The process of changing a Lopez valve daily creates additional work for staff, and staff faces a fear of splash and/or loss of access when it is changed. Staff wanted to know why it needed to be changed daily and if this requirement could be decreased or eliminated. The team found no information in the literature on this type of valve.

Further investigation found a product literature brochure that did not specify or recommend when the device should be changed. The unit protocol specified that the device required changing every 24 hours. The team discussed the EBP findings with the Hospital Epidemiology and Infection Control Department. Nurses were advised to leave the standard as is because the longer the device stayed on the nasogastric tube tip, the more likely it was to become tightly affixed to the tip making it crusty and difficult to separate from the tube. In addition, if the valve was not changed, it posed an infection-control risk of harboring bacteria. In the absence of literature presenting evidence to the contrary, the group decided to continue current practice.

Barriers to EBP

A discussion of the path to translation is not complete without reference to barriers. As with any new policy, program, or initiative, you can anticipate barriers to change. Even if an organization is amenable to innovation and creativity, staff might not be ready or willing to assimilate a particular EBP recommendation. Effective implementation requires a receptive climate and a good fit between the recommended practice change and the users' needs and values (Titler, 2007).

EBP teams must identify barriers to implementation before any efforts at translation can succeed. These barriers can include the following:

- Lack of synergy between behavior of leaders, front-line staff, and other professionals related to EBP (Rapp, Etzel-Wise, Marty, Coffman, Carlson et. al., 2009)

- Difficulty interpreting findings and applying them to practice (Vanhook, 2009)

- Cost and resources required to implement

- Lack of time

- Extrapolation of findings to various groups/populations

- Downstream impact on other processes within the organization

You need to consider if the change is going to improve clinical outcomes, patient or nurse satisfaction, or clinical processes, systems, or operations. Successful implementation of practice change is more likely to occur when the practice change can improve one or more of these factors.

Getting evidence into practice is complex and does not follow a prescribed, logical, or linear path. Evidence, context, and facilitation are key elements in moving evidence into practice. When evidence is disseminated, cultural, social, and/or historical barriers play a role in how the evidence is perceived and whether it is accepted. Contextual or organizational fit and resources available to implement change have been found to be potent predictors of successful implementation of evidence into practice (Rycroft-Malone, Harvey, Seers, Kitson, McCormack et al., 2004).

Teams need to acknowledge the range of diversity of stakeholders and the positive and negative role these individuals and/or teams might play in affecting change.

Professional networks can play a role in the acceptance of change. If a professional organization sponsors the change through practice guidelines, organizations have more support for implementing change. Having a facilitator or project leader can help to move evidence into practice as well. The facilitator has the background and context behind an EBP project and can articulate issues and develop effective implementation strategies. The facilitator is also available to evaluate measures of success (Rycroft-Malone et al. 2004).

Decoding Resistance to Change

To tailor interventions to overcome barriers to change, the team must first assess what is causing the gap between current practice and a specific evidence-based practice. Resistance to change is common and to be expected. Resistance is a form of feedback teams can use to keep dynamic and vibrant conversation about the project alive. After a recommendation for change has been made, the EBP team focuses on reducing resistance to change, viewing resistance as a resource rather than a barrier. Ultimately, a better project implementation plan results if all the identified barriers are noted and the team devises a plan to mitigate these barriers.

A team can use even a litany of complaints or a highly charged conversation to improve the project implementation plan. Change theory and motivational theory are especially helpful in decoding resistance. If resistance is viewed in a positive way and considered as feedback rather than opposition, team members can remain less frustrated in their mission and stay motivated to continue their efforts. Ford and Ford (2009) propose five strategies for decoding resistance to change:

1. Boost awareness (communicate what)

2. Return to purpose (communicate why)

3. Change the change (get it right by capitalizing on feedback)

4. Build participation and engagement (embrace concerns)

5. Complete the past (acknowledge historical failures and turn to the future)

Case in Point

Translating Safe Sleep Evidence into Nursing Practice

Infants who sleep on their backs in a safe sleep environment decrease their risk of dying suddenly and unexpectedly (American Academy of Pediatrics (AAP), 2000, 2005). One component of the safe sleep effort is the "Back to Sleep" Campaign that has halved the number of babies dying from Sudden Infant Death Syndrome (SIDS) (AAP, 2005). This simple intervention is supported by a substantial body of evidence (Dwyer, 2009). The practice adds neither expense nor hardship for parents and communities, yet is inconsistently adopted.

Strategies that accelerate adoption of safe sleep guidelines promise to save lives and move the nation closer to attaining the goals of Healthy People 2020. The Infant Safe Sleep Program (ISSP) was implemented in urban Michigan hospitals and depended on the hospital's ability to develop nursing practice policy, implement policy, and evaluate compliance with policy. The approach provides a model for effective translation of evidence into nursing practice, which applies strategies for decoding of resistance and program evaluation. Results are based on a 4-year project, 2004–2007. This collaborative effort was initiated by Tomorrow's Child/Michigan SIDS, a public health–funded program that interviews and provides grief support to bereaved mothers. Based on these interviews and national data, this forward-thinking program started ISSP.

Collaborative Effort

Building participation and engagement, the ISSP team initiated an extensive collaboration with the target hospitals. They jointly developed clear materials explaining both the desired intervention and the expected outcomes and produced detailed policies and procedures to assure fidelity to the intervention. Nursing policy included both nurse behavior and patient education. The ISSP team provided assistance throughout implementation and evaluation to help address challenges encountered throughout the implementation process.

A process description, including observation and a pre-test/post-test design, answers the following questions: "What is the process to translate evidence on safe sleep into nursing practice in urban Michigan hospitals? Does implementation of a comprehensive approach to safe sleep result in nurses disseminating and role modeling safe sleep messages to parents?"

Tomorrow's Child/Michigan SIDS staff worked with administrators and nurse educators at the hospitals to establish quality improvement processes. Each hospital formed a quality improvement workgroup for infant safe sleep that met regularly for the duration of the ISSP. Tomorrow's Child/Michigan SIDS staff attended workgroup meetings to assist in initiating the project activities and to provide guidance.

Model Policy Development

Each workgroup identified policies that affect newborns and their mothers. The workgroups were charged with reviewing and revising their hospital's policies to include infant safe sleep in clinical practices and information on infant safe sleep in their patient education materials. Model policies were developed. The time between first meeting with hospital staff to final evaluation ranged from 6 to 12 months.

None of the hospitals had policies that met the two sets of criteria for adequate infant safe sleep practice. Each hospital drafted model policies that were adopted after substantial review and discussion with hospital administration. The average time from initiation of project to final crib audit with parent interview ranged from 6 to 12 months. Adoption of safe sleep was a shorter process when hospital administrators were included early in the process. The dedication of both nurse educators and administrative staff was imperative for success. All levels of administration within hospitals needed to be aware and committed to the implementation of the program. Representation at each level of administration was necessary to champion the initiative and to provide continuity to project activities, especially when personnel changed. Hospitals that involved hospital administration at the beginning of the process had a faster adoption of the new policies. Some hospitals already had components of the safe sleep message and expanded existing policy/procedures.

Success

The program was effective. Hospitals involved saw a significant increase in the mean number of safe sleep practices identified by nurses following the education program [t (623) = -8.54, p = .001].

Nurses were asked their opinion on the safest sleep position for an infant and then asked what the AAP recommended as the safest sleep position. Following the educational program, significantly more nurses reported that back was safest as recommended by AAP.

A total of 1,296 cribs were audited pre-policy change, and 1,443 cribs were audited 12 months after the new policies were implemented. Among infants in those cribs at the time of the audits, auditors found a significant increase in the percentage of infants on their backs. They also found a significant increase in the percentage of mothers who had been told about infant safe sleep from 62.7% to 91.4%.

Success in translation of research into practice is multifaceted. All levels of administration within hospitals must be aware of and committed to the implementation of these initiatives. Organizations that identify a person at each level of administration to champion the initiative are more likely to maintain continuity of project activities when staff change. The dedication of both nurse educators and administrative staff is imperative for success. The next challenge is to sustain the program. Sustainability of clinical practice changes is likely because of the organizational culture of these hospitals. Safe sleep training becomes a part of annual competency requirements for nurses.

Adoption of new evidence is a challenging process that requires time. Stakeholder engagement and commitment is an essential and significant facilitator to the process. Sustained clinical practice changes involve both institutional stakeholders and community agencies. This translation program demonstrates that collaboration between agencies results in parents' knowledge of safe sleep for their newborn babies. Nurses facilitate this change by changing nursing policy and implementing safe sleep messages by word and example. Ultimately, this results in saving infant lives.

Acknowledgements: This project was supported by a grant from the Skillman Foundation #2003-352 to Tomorrow's Child/Michigan SIDS.

Conclusion

Many pathways to translation exist. The nature of the evidence is the focal link to translational decision making. This chapter provides translation decision-making guidance for four typical EBP outcomes: compelling evidence, good and consistent evidence, good but conflicting evidence, and insufficient evidence. It also summarizes clinician and environmental barriers to implementation. Evidence is presented as the core of an EBP project. Consideration of the nature of evidence and potential barriers to implementation of change is an important driver of successful translation of EBP into practice. Recommended practice changes must support a good fit among internal and external factors to ensure a smooth translation decision.

References

Adams, S., & Titler, M.G. (2009). Building a learning collaborative. *Worldviews on Evidence-based Nursing.* Oct. 5 [epub ahead of print], pp. 1–9.

American Academy of Pediatrics (AAP). (2005). The changing concept of sudden infant death syndrome: Diagnostic coding shifts, controversies regarding the sleeping environment, and new variables to consider in reducing risk. *Pediatrics, 116*(5), pp. 1245–1255.

American Academy of Pediatrics (AAP). (2000). Task Force on Infant Sleep Position and Sudden Infant Death Syndrome. Changing concepts of sudden infant death syndrome: Implications for infant sleeping environment and sleep position. *Pediatrics, 105*, pp. 650–656.

Center for Disease Control. (2009). Web-based Injury Statistics Query and Reporting System (WISQARS). Retrieved September 22, 2009, from http://www.cdc.gov/injury/wisqars/index.html.

Curley, M. A. Q., Harris, S. K. Fraser, K. A., Johnson, R. A., & Arnold, J. A. (2006). State Behavioral Scale (SBS): A sedation assessment instrument for infants and young children supported on mechanical ventilation. *Pediatric Critical Care Medicine, 7*(2), pp. 107-114.

Dwyer, T. (2009). Sudden infant death syndrome and prone sleeping position. *Annals of Epidemiology, 19*(4), pp. 245–249

Ely, E. W., Truman, B., Shintani, A., Thomason, J. W. W., Wheeler, A. P., Gordon, S. et al. (2003). Monitoring sedation status over time in ICU patients: Reliability and validity of the Richmond Agitation-Sedation Scale (RASS). *Journal of the American Medical Association, 289*(22), pp. 2983–2991.

Ford, J. D., & Ford, L. W. (2009). Decoding resistance to change. *Harvard Business Review, 87*(4), pp. 99–103.

Hidecker, M. J., Jones, R. S., Imig, D. R., & Villarruel, F. A. (2009). Using family paradigms to improve evidence-based practice. *American Journal of Speech-Language Pathology, 18*(3): pp. 212–221.

Hill, K. (2009). Don't lose sight of the importance of the individual in effective falls prevention interventions. *BMC Geriatrics, 9,*: p. 13.

ISMP. (2009). Independent double-checks are vital, not perfect. *ISMP Medication Safety Alert. Nurse Advise-ERR,* 7(2), p. 1.

Li, L. C., Grimshaw, J. M., Nielsen, C., Judd, M., Coyte, P. C., & Graham, I. D. (2009). Use of communities of practice in business and health care sectors: A systematic review. *Implementation Science* 4, p. 27.

McGraw-Hill Companies. (2002). *McGraw-Hill concise dictionary of modern medicine.* New York: author.

Newhouse, R., Dearholt, S., Poe, S., Pugh, L., & White, K. (2007). *Johns Hopkins nursing: Evidence-based practice model and guidelines* (1st ed.). USA: Sigma Theta Tau International.

Nolan, P. & Bradley, E. (2008). Evidence-based practice: Implications and concerns. *Journal of Nursing Management, 16*(4): pp. 388–393.

Ramsay, M. A. E., Savege, T. M., Simpson, B. R. J., & Goodwin, R. (1974). Controlled sedation with alphaxalone-alphadolone. *British Medical Journal, 2*, pp. 656–659.

Rapp, C. A., Etzel-Wise, D., Marty, D., Coffman, M., Carlson, L., Asher, D., Callaghan, J., & Holter, M. (2009). Barriers to evidence-based practice implementation: Results of a qualitative study. *Community Mental Health Journal, 46,* (2).

Rycroft-Malone, J., Harvey, G, Seers, K, Kitson, A, McCormack B, Titchen, A. (2004). An exploration of the factors that influence the implementation of evidence into practice. *Journal of Clinical Nursing, 13*, pp. 913–924.

Timmons, F. & McCabe, C. (2005). How to conduct an effective literature search. *Nursing Standard, 20*(11), pp. 41–47.

Titler, M. (2007). Translating research into practice. *American Journal of Nursing, 107* (6, supplement), pp. 26–33; quiz p. 33.

Vanhook, P. M. (2009). Overcoming the barriers to EBP. *Nursing Management, 40*(8), pp. 9–11.

Applying Translation Science to Improve Health Outcomes

Moving research into clinical practice is not easy. The time required to translate new findings into practice has been estimated at about 17 years (Westfall, Mold, & Fagnan, 2007). Recognizing this difficulty, the National Institutes of Health (NIH) have funded and established a consortium to support this process. Working together, national members share a common vision to improve human health by transforming the research and training environment. This group has been developed to foster the development of a new discipline, Clinical and Translational Science (CTS). Its goal is to use the NIH road map to help translate bench research to clinical practice and back. Consortium members are expected to serve as magnets that concentrate translational and clinical investigators, community clinicians, clinical practices, networks, professional societies, and industry to facilitate the development of new professional interactions, programs, and research projects. Details about these efforts can be accessed electronically (NIH, 2009).

The science base for implementing evidence-based practices (EBPs) continues to be developed. In her groundbreaking report, Titler (2004) suggested that the study of natural experiments would advance the field of translation science. She argued that we need to move beyond describing barriers and facilitators of translating EBP and design research to test interventions that target these barriers. Thus, testing implementation of EBPs in diverse settings begins building a foundation of translation science (Titler, 2004). This chapter explores frameworks and factors that should be considered by practitioners and researchers as components of the translational process.

Framework for Translation

The impact of research and EBP on a cost-restrained, regulated health care environment presents a translation challenge. Rogers (1995) proposed the classic Diffusion of Innovation framework that provides a comprehensive approach to adoption of innovations. Diffusion is a process by which an innovation is communicated over time among members of a social system. Rogers found four primary elements in diffusion:

1. Innovation is an idea or practice that is considered new by an adopting unit including individuals, organizations, or whole health care systems.

2. Communication channels provide the means by which messages are transmitted from one individual to another. Communication can be through formal organizational mechanisms, for example, newsletters, or via informal channels, such as colleagues who socialize together.

3. Time is often critical if the innovation involves implementing a standard or practice to secure the health system's future. The time involved in adopting an innovation can be dependent on the characteristics of the innovation, such as simplicity, trialibility, and observability.

4. Social system is defined as a "set of interrelated units that are engaged in joint problem-solving to accomplish a common goal" (Rogers, 1995, p. 23).

The diffusion pattern has four key drivers or determinants:

1. Alignment of the external environment

2. Features of the adopting organization

3. Features of the innovation

4. Dissemination strategy (Bradley, Webster, Baker, Schlesinger, Inouye et al., 2004; Bradley, Curry, Ramanadhan, Rowe, Nembhard et al., 2009)

Figure 9.1 identifies the major components of each driver.

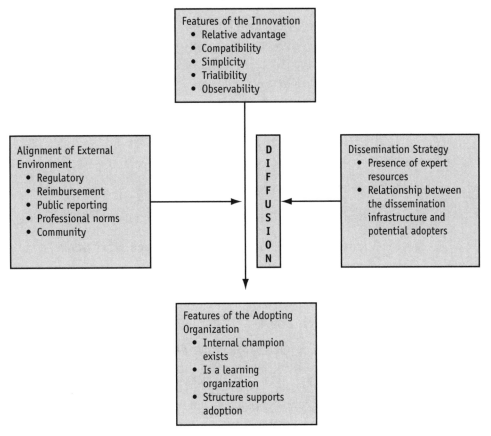

Figure. 9.1: Determinants of Diffusion Pattern

Adapted from Bradley et al., 2009; Bradley et al., 2004

Alignment of External Environment

The Johns Hopkins Nursing EBP (JHNEBP) Model recognizes the influence of external factors on translation of evidence. The external factors that influence the translation of evidence are regulatory compliance, reimbursement, public reporting, professional norms, and community environment. Each factor is reviewed in the context of current forces that affect practice.

Factor 1: Regulatory Compliance

The Joint Commission (TJC), an accrediting organization for health care systems, has established National Patient Safety Goals (NPSGs). The purpose of the NPSGs is to promote improvements in patient safety. The goals and requirements for compliance are guided by a Sentinel Event Advisory Group. Each year, safety goals are reviewed, revised, and updated when needed after a systematic review of the literature and review of reported sentinel events. A sentinel event is an unexpected occurrence involving death or serious physical or psychological injury, or the risk thereof. Serious injury specifically includes loss of limb or function. The phrase "or the risk thereof" includes any process variation for which a recurrence would carry a significant chance of a serious adverse outcome. Further information on sentinel events, including a guideline for conducting root cause analysis, can be found on the TJC website (TJC, 2009).

Challenging goals include the following:

- Improve the safety of using medications (NPSG 3)

- Reduce the risk of health care-associated infections (NSPG 8)

- Accurately and completely reconcile medications across the continuum of care (NPSG 8)

- Reduce the risk of patient harm resulting from falls (NPSG 9)

- Reduce the risk of influenza and pneumococcal disease in institutionalized older adults (NPSG 10)

Each goal has an impact on nursing practice and is further defined by specific processes, for example, implement best practices or evidence-based guidelines to prevent central line bloodstream infections. Achieving these goals might require the adoption of an innovation within a health care organization.

Factor 2: Reimbursement

The Centers for Medicare and Medicaid Services (CMS) on October 1, 2008, enacted new payment provisions. Medicare is no longer going to reimburse hospitals for a higher paying Diagnosis Related Group (DRG) when specific conditions were not present on admission and could have reasonably been prevented using evidence-based guidelines. These conditions are referred to as *never events*. Eight selected hospital-acquired conditions—including pressure ulcers, falls or trauma resulting in serious injury, and vascular catheter-associated and catheter-associated urinary tract infections—are in the first group of diagnoses. The total Medicare cost for payment for these cases is over $20 billion. Further information can be accessed electronically (CMS, 2009).

Factor 3: Public Reporting

Hospital Compare was created through the efforts of the Centers for Medicare and Medicaid Services (CMS), the U. S. Department of Health and Human Services, and other members of the Hospital Quality Alliance (HQA): Improving Care through Information. Participating hospitals have agreed to submit quality information to Hospital Compare to make public the results. Care processes reported for selected conditions, often referred to as core measures, are recorded as percentages of compliance, for example, the percentage of heart failure patients given discharge instruction or the percentage of heart failure patients given smoking cessation advice/counseling.

Hospital Consumer Assessment of Healthcare Providers and Systems (HCAHPS) is a national survey that asks patients about their experiences during a recent hospital stay. A sample of these questions follows:

- How often did nurses communicate well with patients?
- How often did staff explain about medicines before giving them to patients?
- How often was patients' pain well controlled?

Results from each participating hospital are reported in percentages and can be viewed by accessing the Hospital Compare website (U. S. Department of Health and Human Services, 2009).

Factor 4: Professional Norms

Oncology nursing offers an excellent example of application of EBP to oncologic patient care. The Oncology Nursing Society (ONS) Outcomes Resource Area (ORA) provides information for both the nurse providing direct patient care and the nurse who is looking for research evidence regarding outcomes. Evidence-based literature summaries of specific conditions can be found to explain best practices (ONS, 2009).

A major portion of the ORA is devoted to ONS Putting Evidence into Practice (PEP) resources. This area displays tables listing levels of evidence regarding interventions for nursing-sensitive patient outcomes, findings from synthesized reviews or meta-analysis, summaries of relevant guidelines, definitions, and extensive reference lists. All resources on the ORA can be printed from PDF files. Subjects include prevention of infection with evidence rating categories including recommended for practice, likely to be effective, benefits balanced with harms, effectiveness not established, effectiveness unlikely, and not recommended for practice.

American Association of Critical-Care Nurses (AACN) Standards are authoritative statements that describe the level of care and performance common to the profession of nursing by which the quality of nursing practice can be judged. Standards of Care and Standards for Professional Performance for acute and critical care nurses can be accessed on the professional association website (AACN, 2009).

Resources such as these promote evidence-based care and also advocate for the nurse's professional responsibility to be aware of professional association–endorsed guidelines in his or her practice area. Multiple publications outlining scope and standards covering general nursing and a wide array of specialty practices, such as cardiovascular, home health, hospice and palliative, and public health are available from the American Nurses Association (2009).

Factor 5: Community Environment: Health of the Population

The Institute of Medicine's publication *The Future of the Public's Health in the 21ˢᵗ Century* discusses the role of the news media as a powerful tool to direct the public's attention to health issues (2003).

Media tools that promote health behaviors include *social marketing*, which combines marketing influence with social theories to motivate individuals to change behaviors. The diffusion of innovation theory has been used to encourage safe health practices, for example, prevention of sexually transmitted diseases. Nelson provided this compelling message as an example of social marketing math: Every weekend, more than 16,000 children are infected with a sexually transmitted disease. Using numbers and time that people can relate to provides a "hook" to the message (Nelson, 2002).

Compelling messages are ideas that "stick," that is, the ideas are understood and remembered and have an impact that changes the audience's behavior (Heath & Heath, 2007). The Institute for Healthcare Improvement (IHI) 100,000 lives campaign was successful using public media with a message that was "sticky," targeting six EBP areas that had demonstrated improved outcomes. Details of the campaign can be found electronically (IHI, 2006).

Rogers (1995) notes that mass media (radio, television, newspapers) can reach large audiences rapidly, create knowledge, and spread information. Change can also occur if views opposing the new knowledge are not strong and if attitudes are flexible to new ideas. Nurses might be questioned by patients and families about the latest trend or health care innovation reported in the public media, creating pressure for caregivers to remain up-to-date with changes in their area of practice.

Features of the Adopting Organization

According to Bradley and colleagues (2009), adopting organizations have these features:

- Presence of internal champions
- Learning organization environment
- Structural supports

When these features are aligned, translation is enabled.

Internal Champions

Internal champions are critical for diffusion of innovation in adopting organizations. Senior leaders cannot carry the entire burden for diffusion of change. They are, however, in a unique position to be visionary, articulate their vision, and identify key clinical leaders who can serve as internal champions. Ideally, these champions possess clinical expertise, teamwork skills, and communication skills to ignite change diffusion. They have talent in delegating appropriate work to a taskforce or workgroup with appropriate resources.

Successful champions in a clinical setting are ideally practicing clinicians, supplemented by information technology resources and other clinical experts whose skills match the project requirements to maximize success of the team. Champions might be members of the actual workgroup or might be engaged later when the innovation is almost ready for implementation. The role of the champions should be clear with expected time requirements understood and accepted by the champion. Champions might be key clinical leaders by any title, but are often opinion leaders who can help predict and overcome resistance at the local and organizational level.

Learning Organization

Bradley and colleagues (2009) describe organizational use of "positive deviance" as a method that goes beyond performance improvement, assessing best practices in the area of concern and encouraging the organization to learn to apply best practices to its own setting. Adapting these best practices is easiest when organizations share information on practices. Certainly, this sharing is not always a reality in the competitive health care market, but sometimes practices can be identified by formal inquiry to the organization, participation in a collaborative, professional networking, or via the literature. Incentives to adopt best practices might be mandated via regulatory means and public reporting, thus providing high motivation for improvements. Bradley and colleagues (2009) identify steps in the positive deviance approach (see Table 9.1).

Table 9.1: Steps in Positive Deviance Approach

1. Identify the positive deviants or highly performing organizations in your topic of interest.

2. Use qualitative methods; generate a hypothesis about the organization's practices, structure, leadership, culture, and norms that might interact to facilitate high performance.

3. Test your hypothesis via a larger sample of representative highly performing organizations in your industry.

4. Work with stakeholders to convey information learned about best practices. Be aware that each organization provides unique variables that can interact to produce mere mediocrity or great success.

Structural Supports

An adopting organization also must have sufficient structural supports in place for adoption. These supports include data and resources. Bradley (2004) identified several key lessons learned about diffusing innovation into practice. She stated "that data to support start-up, implementation, and ongoing evaluation must be credible and persuasive to those who influence budget decisions" (2004, p.2). Without data, an organization can implement only broad theoretical changes and hope for improvement. With specific pre-and-post measures with supporting graphs, organizations can clearly show progress and the need for modifications to the adopted change. Ideally, ongoing data should be shared with people closest to the work to be changed to engage them in the process and to seek their own ideas to make the adoption process better. Aggregate data should be reported to senior leaders who oversee the success of the innovation. Senior leaders cannot shoulder the entire burden for change, but they can provide the necessary human resource structure for diffusion of changes.

The importance of human resources is often underestimated whenever diffusion of change is needed. Organizations need individuals who can challenge the status quo, people who select individual workgroup members, arrange meetings, write computer programs, gather data, analyze and display findings, make compelling arguments for change, and communicate findings in a positive, motivating manner to front-line workers and upper administration. Preferably, all steps are supplemented with informal networking and interpersonal support that keeps diffusion of change on target, motivating, and enjoyable.

Case in Point

Improving Door-to-Balloon Time after Acute Myocardial Infarction

An example of applying change in a learning organization involves improvement of the core measure for acute myocardial infarction (MI), specifically door-to-balloon time—that is, the time from hospital entry to the start of angioplasty. A large inner-city organization's quality leaders and cardiac interventional laboratory or "cath lab" leaders were not happy with its below national norm scores for door-to-balloon time. Despite having excellent clinicians and low mortality, this group felt challenged by external regulatory mandates and the organization's own competitive culture to improve its score on this measure.

The organization's score calculation was compounded by a low denominator for MI patients included for this core measure. Additionally, some MI patients walked into the emergency department (ED) without prior notice or were transferred from other organizations, thus eliminating precious lead time minutes. The target core measure performance is less than or equal to 90 minutes.

Exploring Changes

The group applied learning organization principles, explored positive deviants, trialed best practices, and monitored data. All organizations must work across groups; the interventional laboratory was challenged by different departments, multiple leaders who reported to different directors, and a busy ED with many trauma cases. When examining positive deviants, the group found that in some highly performing organizations, emergency medical personnel phone ahead to the ED about a confirmed ST-elevation MI. Other organizations with outstanding scores had personnel who were cross-trained or in geographically close proximity to the ED and the cath lab or to the cardiac care unit (CCU) and the cath lab. This cross-training or proximity allowed a trained clinician to alert the cath lab team and initiate prep procedures for the interventional case.

Diffusion of change must apply qualitative methods and hypothesis testing. The cath lab multidisciplinary team examined data, reviewed outliers that negatively affected their scores, explored positive deviants, and considered what they could do to apply similar but unique procedures.

Implementing Changes

The team implemented the following actions:

- Made use of early alert notification, engaging the ED to work with emergency medical services for alerts to possible ST elevation MIs.

- Assured necessary blood work was drawn stat and 12-lead ECG taken in the ED.

- Worked with ED physician leaders to have the ED physician read and verify the ECG findings.

- Administered medications in the ED per cardiology best practice guidelines.

- Designated a single room and one alternate room in the cath lab to use for on-call MI cases, stocking the room appropriately and labeling vital equipment.

- Educated targeted individuals in cath lab specifics (room setup, medication, monitoring equipment, emergency equipment, and so on).

- To minimize travel time delays, identified cath lab clinicians who lived the closest to the hospital (less than 30 minutes away) so that these individuals could be on call for cases.

- Utilized critical care transporters to transfer the patient from the ED directly to the cath lab and begin the prep process while the cath lab on-call team was coming to the hospital.

- Introduced team members who would likely be working together during cases.

- Set up data collection methods for the following time entries: arrival at door, ECG, ED physician ECG reading, ED physician activation of emergency transport team, arrival of patient into the cath lab, start of balloon procedure, and total time from door to balloon.

- Conducted a multidisciplinary review of all ST-elevation myocardial infarction cases within 48 hours to identify areas of improvement.

Group Dynamics and Results

Project leaders had to work with stakeholders and assign champions. Champions of each of the involved departments (ED, critical care transport team, cath lab, cardiac care unit, and interventional cardiology) had to be aware of the rationale for trialing a different method. These individuals met every week for a year and then decreased meeting frequency to every other week to monitor individual case data, offer improvement ideas, and modify practice as needed. The group challenged workplace cultures as they continued to work toward a common cause. The multiple departmental priorities had to be coalesced into a common goal. The group was challenged by the fact that each department had a different work focus. While the cath lab focused on the interventional cardiology specialty, the ED's focus was general emergency medicine, triage, and disposition of patients with multiple bodily system maladies. Additionally, the cath lab staff was acutely sensitive to ST-elevation myocardial infarctions, while the ED staff performed and read many ECGs on a given shift during the performance of multiple lab tests and X-ray work and were less sensitive to ST changes. Thirdly, the cath lab was focused on prompt treatment, while the ED was focused on emergency medicine while assessing the need to admit or discharge its patients. Only one of the dispositions of the ED would be to the cath lab. The group discovered that they could best approach the work by agreeing on what they had in common—emergency treatment of a cardiac condition to quickly isolate that subset of patients and move them efficiently along the care continuum to the cath lab. That focus met the needs of both groups.

The group celebrated success and excellent compliance scores; they viewed disappointments as learning opportunities. One year post-intervention, outcomes showed that the time to balloon improved by 44%. The multidisciplinary group, in its continual efforts to achieve best practice, has recently raised their goal to a desired 95% compliance with this core measure.

Innovation

Rogers (1995) identifies specific characteristics of the innovation that contribute to its adoption and speed of adoption: relative advantage, compatibility, complexity, trialibility, and observability. This section uses an example from a patient unit that focuses on care of patients diagnosed with Human Immunodeficiency Virus (HIV) to discuss these characteristics.

The impact of widespread social marketing campaigns disseminating HIV awareness and prevention messages is minimal without a system of targeting smaller groups of vulnerable individuals, the factors that contribute to health literacy, and the abilities of those individuals to alter their own determinants of health. In addition to findings in the literature, staff on an inpatient unit that cares for predominately HIV patients has reported through observation that low literacy levels among the primary patient population admitted to the service likely interferes with comprehension of complex medication regimens, follow-up, and health maintenance programs. Nurses attribute recidivism, poor health outcomes, and nonadherence with treatment regimens to the low literacy and lack of available resources for both providers and patients to intervene. The nurses on the patient care unit were concerned about their patient's understanding and compliance with the highly active antiretroviral therapy (HAART) regimen. They decided to intervene by supplementing patient education with visual tools and teach-back methods to improve understanding of their medications. Teach-back is a method to enhance understanding by asking individuals to explain the information that has been discussed in their own words.

The innovation is incorporating the teach-back method with a standardized medication teaching tool that provides color pictures of each medication used in the HAART regimen. Teach-back is reportedly a method that achieves understanding in the informed consent process (Kripalani, Bengtzen, Henderson, & Jacobson, 2008). The application of the characteristics of innovations defined by Rogers (1995) and updated by Bradley (2009) is depicted in Table 9.2.

Table 9.2: Application of the Characteristics of Innovations

Characteristic and/or Definition	Application to Intervention
Relative advantage: The perception that an innovation is better than the idea it precedes.	Will the individual patients perceive an advantage to having consistent information provided and being asked to repeat back the information to the nurse? Is the nursing staff willing to commit the time to adopt this new method of patient education? The patients can receive their medications without cost through outpatient follow-up at a hospital clinic.
Compatibility: The degree to which an innovation is consistent with existing values, past experiences, and the needs of the adopters.	In this example, the adopters are both the nurses and patients on the unit. The nurses are familiar with the drug regimens the patients are using; however, they have concern that the observed nonadherence might be in part related to literacy.
Simplicity: The ability of an innovation to be understood and used.	The nurses have developed a scripted teaching tool that discusses each medication, dose, and possible side effects that a patient might experience. A brief measure of literacy, Rapid Estimate of Adult Literacy in Medicine (REALM) was added to the admission nursing assessment (Davis, Long, Jackson, Mayeaux, George, Murphy et al., 1993). Do the members of the social system understand the purpose for the innovation? The nurses see recidivism as an issue in their patients. The standard medication information is meant to simplify complex medication therapies.
Trialibility: The degree to which an innovation might be experimented on a limited basis.	Laminated HAART charts are readily available for education. Before discharge, the patients are shown how to fill a weekly pill container with their actual medications.
Observability: The ability to view the results of the innovation.	Patient outcomes can be measured by disease progression, readmissions, lower CD4 counts, and higher viral loads that might indicate nonadherence. Patient satisfaction can be assessed with a focus on discharge preparation and patient knowledge of medications. Literacy levels can be correlated with recidivism and time to achieve teach-back.

A national initiative sponsored by IHI and The Robert Wood Johnson Foundation is testing many innovations identified by medical-surgical bedside caregivers. The IHI initiative "Transforming Care at the Bedside (TCAB)" is an example of innovations designed and trialed in patient care areas, ranging from white boards that designate when a nurse is able to take an admission to van rides home for patients (IHI, 2004).

Dissemination Strategy

Diffusion occurs within a social system. Many innovations are conceptualized through small pilot projects, often within a larger organization. The IHI published a white paper making suggestions for preparing for spread (2004). The IHI sees spread as a leadership responsibility after the innovation demonstrates the innovation to be clearly better than current state. Needed elements for dissemination include a communication strategy using a clear message by people who are capable of influencing others in the target population. Although the IHI (2004) brings improvement teams together, as in the TCAB project, the spread of the innovation is in the domain of an organization's senior leadership. Resources such as staff time might be required as part of the innovation. Recognition by senior leaders that resources are required for diffusion can ensure strategies of implementation are not thwarted.

Bradley and colleagues (2004) characterized the dissemination as requiring two essentials components:

1. Presence of expert resources for ongoing dissemination efforts to clinicians and administrators

2. Relationship between the dissemination infrastructure and the potential adopters

Great ideas come from bedside caregivers in an organization. Champions are thought of as engines of change; however, a small improvement team led by champions cannot be solely responsible to spread innovations within an organization. The role of the teams is to test the innovation and serve as experts to explain new innovations to potential adopters (Bodenheimer, 2007).

Rogers' division of adopters of innovations into groups that form a bell curve is widely accepted. The range of innovation adoption is from the *innovators* who develop an innovation to the last ones who join in the change, known as *the laggards.* The first two groups, the *innovators* and *early adopters* are considered as visionaries bringing new ideas and innovations to practice (Gladwell, 2000). The next group, *early majority*, represent about one-third of the adopters in the framework (Rogers, 1995). Members of this group are those open to new ideas but are also tasked with the application of new best practices. Finding these individuals in the organization is critical to the adoption of an innovation and they should be used as the pilot unit. Once the effort is embraced and implementation begins there is a point when the innovation is recognized as being an improvement and becomes widely accepted and adopted, which Gladwell (2000) characterized as the "tipping point." After this occurs the next group, the *late majority,* are beginning to recognize and incorporate the improvement. The last group, the *laggards*, are traditionalists slow to adopt but may provide stability to an organizational unit in turbulent times. For front-line caregivers, an innovation affecting their daily work must be seen as a clear advantage, for example, improvement on publicly reported measures of direct care. Bodenheimer (2007) notes that concerns from those individuals working daily to care for patients must be heard and not considered as laggards in the adoption of changes.

Champions, as frequent users and problem solvers, provide a resource to disseminate the innovation to other clinicians and administrators. Local champions should develop a toolkit to help with innovation spread. The IHI provides 21 implementation toolkits at their website (IHI, n.d.).

In complex organizations, choosers of innovations might not be the users (Dearing, 2008). Process innovations cause change in the workflow; however, the work environment might also need adjustment. Although practitioners might want to modify innovations to create a "better fit," Dearing suggests adopters should modify a process or program by adding local components. This addition can help the adopters avoid deleting components of the process that are essential to the effectiveness of the innovation. "Guided adaption" serves to explain to adopters what aspects of a process are essential for the effect to be achieved and what components are possibly changeable (Dearing, 2008). Using Dearing's suggestions, adaptation becomes part of the adoption process, and fidelity becomes an outcome property. Fidelity is defined as the degree to which program adopters implement programs as intended by the originators (Rohrbach, Grana, Sussman, & Valente, 2006).

Innovation-Decision Process

A key message is the realization that health care innovations must reduce costs to be sustainable. An organization paying for an innovation must derive benefit, or that organization is going to find it difficult to sustain the innovation. Many transitional care programs facilitating the movement of patients from hospital to community have demonstrated excellent pilot results (Coleman, Parry, Chalmers, & Min, 2006; Jack, Chetty, Anthony, Greenwald, Sanchez et al., 2009). Hospitals using personnel resources to provide the innovation must align revenue with the expenses to help sustain the innovation.

The decision process by an organization to accept or reject an innovation is complex as illustrated in Figure 9.2.

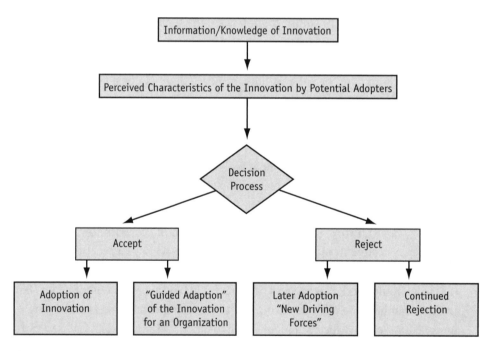

Figure 9.2: Decision Process

Rogers (1995) suggests that the decision could be adoption or rejection. However, health care organizations have unique cultures and the decision is complex even when an innovation is accepted. Adaption may need to occur to ensure fit within the norms of the organization. Bradley and colleagues (2009) illustrated positive deviance as a method that can be used by organization members who are advocates of the innovation. If "guided adaption" is chosen, fidelity of the vital components of the innovation must be used by the adopting organization to ensure outcomes. Rogers notes that initial rejection could be followed later by adoption. Today, payment incentives may be realigned with health reform, and innovations rejected as not cost-effective could be reconsidered as innovative approaches as new driving forces occur in the health care environment. The determinants of diffusion are continuously changing the health care system.

Promoting Action on Research Implementation in Health Services

Kitson, Harvey, and McCormack developed the Promoting Action on Research Implementation in Health Services (PARiHS) framework to facilitate the translation of knowledge (1998). This framework is excellent for outlining the components of innovation adoption with concepts familiar to clinicians. Kitson and colleagues' formula for successful implementation of evidence guidelines or research is a function of three interrelated concepts: evidence, context, and facilitation. A formula to illustrate successful implementation of the framework is

$$SI = f (E, C, F)$$

Successful implementation (SI) is a function (f) of evidence (E), context (C), and facilitation (F).

Evidence

Kitson and colleagues' framework includes research, clinical experiences, and patient preferences in their definition of evidence. They describe a continuum for each of these elements, recognizing that Level I evidence, for example, randomized control trials (RCTs), is at one end of the continuum with anecdotal evidence at the other end. Clinical experience is viewed along a continuum ranging from a high level of consensus to divided expert opinion. Patient preferences are viewed at one end of the spectrum as highly integrated with partnerships between provider and patient or at the other end of the spectrum with no patient involvement.

   In practice, it is typical to find that even Level I evidence of an RCT might not be feasible to implement if clinicians do not find the intervention practical and safe. For example, the gold standard for confirmation of placement of a nasogastric tube for feeding is chest X-ray, but how many times can a patient safely be exposed to X-ray to confirm nasogastric tube placement? Clinicians can adopt supplemental methods to confirm placement of nasogastric tubes, such as colorimetric carbon dioxide testing, by investigating evidence from research literature and nonresearch literature (Burns, Carpenter, Blevins, Bragg, Marshall et al., 2006; Meyer, Henry, Maury, Baudel, Guidet et al., 2009). Therefore, both research and nonresearch evidence is often needed to determine a translation strategy in the clinical environment.

Context

What goes on in adopting organizations can make the difference in the likelihood of positive and intended outcomes being achieved. McCormack, Kitson, Harvey, Rycroft-Malone, Titchen et al. (2002) completed a concept analysis of the meaning of "context." She found three sub-elements contribute to the characteristics of context including culture, leadership, and evaluation. Each sub-element has components to explore when an organization is adopting an innovation into a system:

1. Culture: Type of organization, its cultures and beliefs, collaborative relationships among clinicians who work together

2. Leadership and Management: Listening and responding to staff concerns; resonant leadership that supports nursing practice by providing resources and removing barriers

3. Evaluation: Providing feedback on performance both for individuals and teams; multiple evaluation measures used to evaluate progress including clinical and economic indicators

McCormack and colleagues concluded that the elements within *context* coalesce to either enable change or to act as barriers.

Facilitation

People who make things easier or help others toward achieving goals are facilitators. Kitson and colleagues (1998) distinguish a facilitator from a local opinion leader. An opinion leader informally influences individual behavior. However, in translating research or evidence into practice, the facilitator's role is to help individuals understand what needs to change and how to bring forward the change. Facilitators use a series of skills to achieve change whereas opinion leaders might influence because of their status or technical ability. Opinion leaders can be peers and experts. Facilitators can come from outside an organization, whereas opinion leaders are often found within the system. Locock, Dopson, Chambers, and Gabbay (2001) provide an excellent discussion of the role of opinion leaders.

Facilitators in Action

Alkema and Frey (2006) used the PARiHS framework to translate a Community-Based Medication Management (CBM) Intervention. The original program implemented an evidence-based medication management intervention to reduce medication problems in frail older adults. An expert consensus panel developed home health criteria. These criteria focus on factors that can be assessed by home health nurses and resolved as part of the plan of care. The model was empirically tested by a university with a randomized control trial (Meredith, Feldman, Frey, Hall, Arnold, Brown, & Ray, 2002).

The innovation, an evidence-based program developed from the randomized trial, was implemented in a Medicaid waiver care management program in two different agencies. The intervention centered on having an on-site pharmacist who served as a consultant within the home health care setting to assist nurses in resolving medication problems. Using this model resolved medication problems in 50% of the intervention group compared to 38% of the control group. Three additional outcome measures showed improvement.

Technical assistance facilitated the translation of the CBM Intervention into four additional home health agencies. Within these settings, the model was feasible and sustainable in providing in-home services to the frail elderly. The translation of the program into a different practice environment that serves disabled low-income older adults demonstrated stress between model fidelity and adoption to the new setting. The evidence was strong; however, the context in which the research was placed was different. The model of care included nurses and social workers in the role of primary care managers. The pharmacist was available by phone and occasionally on-site. Occasionally, social workers were placed in the position of contacting the primary physician about medication issues. Staff visitation for the disabled included monthly phone calls and quarterly visits compared to several times a week in the original study. The facilitation team from the first intervention site was on-site specifically for meetings and phone consults. Alkema and Frey (2006) conclude that program evaluation of translation of the CBM intervention needs to capture outcomes at a client level and also the lessons learned by implementing an evidence-based practice in diverse settings.

Partnerships in Translation

Translation of evidence into practice challenges practitioners to evaluate the strength in developing partnerships. These partnerships can take shape between and among researchers and practitioners, health care organizations and schools of nursing, and diverse health care settings.

Researchers and Practitioners

Developing evidence through randomized control trials provides health care practitioners with best practice knowledge. Translation to practice from the "ideal" research setting of controlled trials to "real"-world practices requires an extension of research into diverse contexts. Clinical practitioners can help researchers interpret best practice processes. The term "knowledge brokers" has been used to describe individuals who serve as the link between researchers and the bedside practitioners. Educators and clinical specialists often have the designated organizational role of knowledge broker, assuming the responsibility for translating new evidence into practice (Kent, Hutchinson, & Fineout-Overholt, 2009).

The complexity of health care organizations is best critiqued by those who practice in the setting. Facilitation of organization-wide EBP implementation by either opinion leaders or change agents needs to be completed with an understanding of the organization culture. An example that illustrates this point is an institution's adoption of an institutional vaccination protocol to help meet regulatory compliance. Despite vaccination compliance being an element of an evidence-based core measure reported by the hospital and approved as an institutional vaccination policy for adult patients, implementation across the institution was not smooth. Several departments expressed concerned that vaccination might cause post-vaccination fever, prompting unnecessary and costly work ups and possibly prolonging length of hospitalization. Some departments adopted the policy only because of facilitation by change agents such as performance improvement leaders, educators and physician, and nursing opinion leaders, and because of the scientific evidence provided. Opinion leaders within departments needed to hear the concerns at the local and departmental level, follow-up with answers to those specific concerns, and develop an implementation strategy and timeline. This example stresses the importance of two-way communication whenever a challenging policy is implemented. Just mandating something does not equate to acceptance and implementation. Even today, some departments have chosen alternative methods to meet compliance that are better suited to their patient populations.

Health Care Organizations and Schools of Nursing

Four years of collaboration between nurses at The Johns Hopkins Hospital (JHH) and The Johns Hopkins University School of Nursing (JHUSON) resulted in the synergy of ideas about practice and the development of the JHNEBP Model. This collaboration continues in dissemination of the model and in collaboration in other venues.

At JHH, the Nursing Research Committee with members representing clinical divisions of the hospital includes a faculty member from the JHUSON. Clinical nurse committee members have identified an Art and Nursing Research Study that they want to develop into a research proposal. The study plan uses quantitative (survey) and qualitative (focus groups) measures and is to be a combined proposal from JHH and JHUSON. The JHUSON faculty is assisting the committee to look for a small grant to subsidize the study through the JHUSON Development Office. The faculty member is an expert in conducting focus groups; the hospital nurse researcher has a quantitative research focus. Combining the researchers' and clinicians' expertise results in the ability to conduct a mixed-methods study in the acute care setting. The JHUSON and JHH are each going to disseminate the results from the study evaluating the benefit of incorporating art as a media to reduce stress in practicing nurses and student nurses.

Diverse Settings Partnerships

Best practices can be translated from the site of origination to other settings, including community hospitals, health departments, regulatory agencies, and patient homes. This is referred to as a Type II translation, which is aimed at enhancing the adoption of effective practices in the community (Rohrbach, Grana, Sussman, & Valente, 2006). In the process of translation, identifying community stakeholders is critical for those who disseminate findings and for those who are invested in implementing programs. The dissemination of programs into other settings can employ several techniques.

Rohrbach, Grana, Sussman, and Valente (2006) explored program provider training methodology to enhance adoption and implementation. Techniques ranged from material only, for example, toolkit; to materials plus workshops; to materials, workshops, and technical assistance/consultation for a six-month period. The last and most comprehensive approach was associated with high levels of program adoption and implementation. However, the cost of workshops and consultation can be a barrier to the decision to adopt an innovation. Therefore, an assessment of the dissemination strategy must be coupled with an assessment of the complexity of the innovation. Toolkits with checklists might suffice in adopting an innovation that is easily understandable, such as evidence-based controlling of bloodstream infections through procedure checklists and empowering critical care nurses to stop an insertion if a violation in the protocol occurs (Pronovost, Needham, Berenholtz, Sinopoli, Chu et al., 2006).

Case in-Point

Nurse-Pharmacist Collaboration on Medication Reconciliation

An estimated 400,000 preventable adverse drug events (ADEs) occur in hospitals each year resulting in at least $3.5 billion in extra costs (Institute of Medicine, 2007). A contributing factor of these ADEs is incomplete medication information. In 2005, The Joint Commission (TJC) recognized this problem by establishing a National Patient Safety Goal to promote medication reconciliation. Recognizing the difficulty of completing medication reconciliation, TJC suspended grading of the standard in 2009; however, a revised standard is to be introduced in 2010 (Mansur, 2009).

Practice Question

Does using a nurse-pharmacist team to identify and correct discrepancies during medication reconciliation on admission and discharge reduce the number of medication errors in acute medical patients?

Evidence

Deficits in information transfer across the care continuum place the patient at serious risk for harm (Kripalani, LeFevre, Phillips, Williams, Basaviah & Baker, 2007). Nowhere is this more evident than with respect to the medication use process. Physicians and nurses have historically obtained medication history information; however, the hurried admission process leaves little time to explore a detailed medication history. Organizations have responded to this continuity of care challenge by developing physician-led, nurse-led, and pharmacist-led medication reconciliation processes to prevent harm (Gleason, Groszek, Sullivan, Rooney, Barnard et al., 2004; Cornish, Knowles, Marchesano, Tam, Shadowitz et al., 2005).

Because a literature review yielded little evidence in this practice area, a research study was designed to contribute new information. The study, funded by The Robert Wood Johnson Foundation's Interdisciplinary Nursing Quality Research Initiative (INQRI), was aimed at testing the effectiveness and cost benefit of a nurse-pharmacist team in identifying and correcting unintended discrepancies in acute medical patients during medication reconciliation on admission and discharge. Study findings included the following:

- Of the 563 patients who entered the study, 226 (40%) experienced discrepancies on admission or discharge.

- 162 patients (28%) had discrepancies rated as having the potential to cause harm as determined by two physicians and two pharmacists.

- An average of 11 minutes was required for the study nurse to complete the patient medication interview protocol and an additional 29 minutes to complete the list.

Translation

External Environment

In this era of health reform, strong evidence indicates that Medicare patients return to the hospital within 30 days of discharge at rates of over 19.6% at a cost of $17.4 billion in health care spending (Jencks, Williams, & Coleman, 2009). Payment for care episodes, inclusive of the 30 days after hospital discharge, is being proposed in Congress and is designed to eliminate the payment that now occurs for each admission. Health care organizational responsibility extends into the patients' communities. Assurance of complete medication reconciliation is the key to avoid unplanned re-entry into the system and loss of revenue. Discharge calls or visits by the hospital care team might provide a safety net until the patient can access the primary care provider.

Features of the Innovation

The premise underlying the nurse-pharmacist model was that replication can be achieved by other organizations. Research nurses were clinicians who were involved in bedside care before the study. With knowledge of the hospital systems and structures, the nurses were equipped to implement the study and develop workflow processes. They modified practice from handwritten medication lists to electronic entry of these lists. Pharmacist consultation was facilitated by using a pager system with texted communication.

Use of a nurse-pharmacist team was seen by the bedside care team as providing a relative advantage in that the study team had time to access outside sources of information, for example, community pharmacies. The study team communicated with patients after discharge to correct any discharge discrepancies and provided a wallet-sized medication card, and they used organizational resources to incorporate the innovation into daily operations. Other organizations planning to trial this innovation could use current resources to establish a team or team functions within existing structures. A toolkit might be sufficient because of the simplicity of the innovation.

Features of the Adopting Organization

The team needs to leverage its internal champions, many of whom are involved in the research study. In anticipation of questions and ideas, the team plans for special attendance at select meetings by key study team members. The study site is a learning organization, so showing data that includes harm scores and financial implications can be very compelling. The team shows that the institution indeed can and must do better with medication reconciliation.

The current departmental structure does not easily support adoption. A research nurse spends almost 30 additional minutes to accurately reconcile admission medications. Assessing roles that support patient care, for example, point-of-care pharmacists, case managers, or mid-level providers, might identify opportunities to restructure work and integrate the innovation into existing roles.

Dissemination Strategy

The study has just ended. The team schedules presentations to key groups in the organization, such as safety and quality improvement committees. The research nurses, who have developed expertise in this intervention, have designed a toolkit that explains successful workflow processes. The relationship between the dissemination infrastructure and potential adopters is the biggest challenge. The team must make the regulatory, financial, and moral case to redesign workflow so that medication reconciliation duties at admission and discharge are reassigned to a care provider who has the knowledge and time to complete the process.

The organization is implementing new information systems whose functionality can be leveraged to identify high-risk patients for an enhanced medication reconciliation protocol. New partnerships with home care providers can provide assessment of medication compliance after discharge. A change in payment

structure by Medicare to episodes of care can move the system to develop new strategies and partnerships that can spotlight the need for transitional care quality improvements across all organizations.

Lessons Learned

An evidence-based change in care requires multiple sources of support.

1. Keep key audiences informed during the evidence-based investigation and/or research study. Waiting until all results are analyzed or all the literature is reviewed can result in delayed dissemination. In this example, the study team was aware of the study trends, but they did not brief key leadership decision makers during the study. Although most investigators want to share results at the completion of a project, this can delay adoption.

2. The decision to accept or reject an innovation can change over time. A change in health care payment might stimulate adoption of this innovation. Champions who have knowledge of the innovation and persuasive power are essential to ensure the adoption decision is balanced when compared to the present state.

3. Adoption strategies in a decentralized organization can vary; therefore, the development of a toolkit can help maintain the fidelity of the intervention model.

Summary

This chapter uses the Determinants of Diffusion framework to explore factors that must be considered when translating innovations into practice. Assessment of an organizations readiness to adopt a new practice must be evaluated within the context of the external environment, features of the innovation, the driving forces for change in the adopting organization, and a planned strategy for dissemination. Implementing EBPs in diverse settings builds knowledge and contributes to the foundation of translation science.

References

Alkema, G. E. & Frey, D. (2006). Implications of translating research into practice: A medication management intervention. *Home Health Care Services Quarterly, 25*(1–2), pp. 33–54.

American Association of Critical-Care Nurses. (2009). Standards of care for acute and critical care nursing practice. Retrieved November 13, 2009, from http://classic.aacn.org/AACN/practice.nsf/Files/acstds/$file/130300StdsAcute.pdf

American Nurses Association. (2009). *ANA standards*. Retrieved November 17, 2009, from http://www.nursesbooks.org/Main-Menu/Standards/H--N.aspx

Bodenheimer, T. (2007). The science of spread: How innovations in care become the norm. Retrieved May 21, 2010, from http://www.chef.org/~/media/Files/PDF/T/The ScienceOfSpread.pdf

Bradley, E. H., Curry, L. A., Ramanadhan, S., Rowe, L., Nembhard, I. M., & Krumholz H.M. (2009). Research in action: Using positive deviance to improve quality of health care. *Implementation Science, 4*, p. 25.

Bradley, E. H., Webster, T. R., Baker, D., Schlesinger, M., Inouye, S. K., Barth, M. C., et al. (2004). Translating research into practice: Speeding the adoption of innovative health care programs. *Commonwealth Fund.*

Burns, S. M., Carpenter, R., Blevins, C., Bragg, S., Marshall, M., Browne, L., et al. (2006). Detection of inadvertent airway intubation during gastric tube insertion: Capnography versus a colorimetric carbon dioxide detector. *American Journal of Critical Care, 15*(2), pp. 188–195.

Centers for Medicare and Medicaid Services. (2009). CMS proposes to expand quality program for hospital inpatient services in FY 2009. Retrieved November 13, 2009, from http://www.cms.hhs.gov/apps/media/press/release.asp?Counter=3041

Coleman, E., Parry. C, Chalmers, S. & Min, S. (2006). The care transitions intervention model: Results of a randomized controlled trial. *Archives of Internal Medicine, 166*, pp. 1822–1828.

Cornish, P. L., Knowles, S. R., Marchesano, R., Tam, V., Shadowitz, S., Juurlink, D. N. et al. (2005). Unintended medication discrepancies at the time of hospital admission. *Archives of Internal Medicine, 165*(4), pp. 424–429.

Davis, T. C., Long, S. W., Jackson, R. H., Mayeaux, E. J., George, R. B., Murphy, P. W.,et al. (1993). Rapid estimate of adult literacy in medicine: A shortened screening instrument. *Family Medicine 25*(6), pp. 391–395.

Dearing, J. W. (2008). Evolution of diffusion and dissemination theory. *Journal of Public Health Management and Practice, 14*(2), pp. 99–108.

Gladwell, M. (2000). *The Tipping Point.* New York: Little, Brown and Company.

Gleason, K. M, Groszek, J. M, Sullivan, C., Rooney, D., Barnard, C., Noskin, G. A. et al. (2004). Reconciliation of discrepancies in medication histories and admission orders of newly hospitalized patients. *American Journal of Health System Pharmacists, 61*(16), pp.1689–1695.

Heath, C. & Heath, D. (2007). *Made to stick.* New York: Random House.

Institute for Healthcare Improvement. (2006). Remaking American medicine. Retrieved November 13, 2009, from http://www.remakingamericanmedicine.org/lives.html

Institute for Healthcare Improvement. (n.d.). Retrieved November 13, 2009, from http://www.ihi.org/ihi/search/searchresults.aspx?searchterm=toolkits&pg=1&searchtype= basic

Institute for Healthcare Improvement. (2004). Transforming care at the bedside. Retrieved November 17, 2009, from http://www.rwjf.org/files/publications/other/IHITCABpaper%5B1%5D.pdf

Institute of Medicine. (2003). *The Future of the public's health in the 21st century.* Washington, DC: The National Academies Press.

Institute of Medicine. (2007). *Preventing medication errors.* Washington, DC: The National Academies Press.

Jack, B. W., Chetty, V. K., Anthony, D., Greenwald, J. L., Sanchez, G. M., Johnson, A. E. et al. (2009). A reengineered hospital discharge program to decrease rehospitalization. *Annals of Internal Medicine, 150*, pp. 178–187.

Jencks, S. F., Williams, M. V., & Coleman, E. A. (2009). Rehospitalizations among patients in the Medicare fee-for-service program. *The New England Journal of Medicine, 360*(14), pp. 1418–1428.

The Joint Commission. (2009). National patient safety goals. Retrieved November 13, 2009, from http://www.jointcommission.org/patientsafety/nationalpatientsafetygoals/

Kent, B., Hutchinson, A. M., & Fineout-Overholt, E. (2009). Getting evidence into practice-Understanding knowledge translation to achieve practice change. *Worldview on Evidence-Based Nursing*, 3rd Quarter, 183-185.

Kitson, A., Harvey, G., and McCormack, B. (1998). Enabling the implementation of evidence based practice: a conceptual framework. *Quality in Health Care, 7*, pp. 149–158.

Kripalani, S., Bengtzen, R., Henderson, L.E., & Jacobson, T. A. (2008). Clinical research in low-literacy populations: Using teach-back to assess comprehensive of informed consent and privacy information. *Ethics and Human Research, March-April*, pp. 13–19.

Kripalani, S., LeFevre, F., Phillips, C. O., Williams, M. V., Basaviah, P., & Baker, D. W. (2007). Deficits in communication and information transfer between hospital-based and primary care physicians: Implications for patient safety and continuity of care. *JAMA: The Journal of the American Medical Association, 297*(8), pp. 831–841.

Locock, Dopson, Chambers, & Gabbay. (2001). Understanding the role of opinion leaders in improving clinical effectiveness. *Social Science and Medicine, 53*(6), pp. 745–757.

Mansur, J. M. (2009). A continuing need to reconcile medications for patient safety. *Joint Commission Journal on Quality and Patient Safety, 35*(5), p. 263.

McCormack, B., Kitson, A., Harvey, G., Rycroft-Malone, J., Titchen, A., & Seers, K et al. (2002). Getting evidence into practice: the meaning of 'context'. *Journal of Advanced Nursing, 38*(1), pp. 94–104.

Meredith, S., Feldman, P., Frey, D., Giammarco, L., Hall, K., Arnold, K. et al. (2002). Improving medication use in newly admitted home healthcare patients: a randomized controlled trial. *Journal of the American Geriatrics Society, 50*(9), pp. 1484–1491.

Meyer, P., Henry, M., Maury, E., Baudel, J. L., Guidet, B., & Offenstadt, G.et al. (2009). Colorimetric capnometry to ensure correct nasogastric tube position. *Journal of Critical Care, 24*(2), pp. 231–235.

National Institutes of Health. (2009). Re-engineering the clinical research enterprise. Retrieved November 13, 2009, from http://nihroadmap.nih.gov/clinicalresearch/overview-translational.asp

Nelson, D. (2002). Communicating public health information effectively. In Nelson, D., Brownson, R., Remington, P., Parvanta, C. (Eds.). *Translating Public Health Data.* American Public Health Association: Washington, DC, pp. 33–45.

Oncology Nursing Society. (2009). Evidence-Based Practice Resource Area (EBPRA). Retrieved November 13, 2009, from http://onsopcontent.ons.org/toolkits/evidence/

Pronovost, P., Needham, D., Berenholtz, S., Sinopoli, D., Chu H, Cosgrove, S., et al. (2006). An intervention to decrease catheter-related bloodstream infections in the ICU. *New England Journal of Medicine, 355*(26), pp. 2725–2732.

Rogers, E. M. (1995). *Diffusion of innovations.* New York: The Free Press.

Rohrbach, L. A., Grana, R., Sussman, S., & Valente, T. W. (2006). Type II translation: Transporting prevention interventions from research to real-world settings. *Evaluation and the Health Professions, 29*(3), pp. 302–333.

Titler, M. G. (2004). Methods in translation science. *Worldviews on Evidence-Based Nursing, 1,* pp. 38–48.

U. S. Department of Health and Human Services. (2009). *Hospital Compare* - A quality tool provided by Medicare. Retrieved April 9, 2010 from http://www.hospitalcompare.hhs.gov/Hospital/Search/SearchMethod.asp?pagelist=Home&dest=NAV|Home|Search|SearchMethod|Welcome&search_dest=NAV|Home|Search|Welcome&version=default&browser=Firefox|3|WinXP&language=English&btnFindHosp=Find+and+Compare+

Westfall, J. M., Mold, J., & Fagnan, L. (2007). Practice-Based Research—Blue highways on the NIH roadmap. *JAMA: The Journal of the American Medical Association, 297*(4), pp. 403–406.

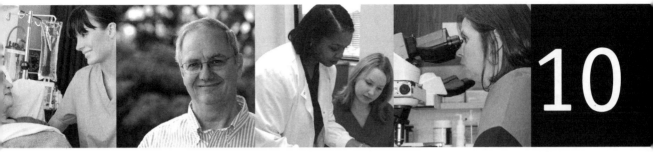

Translating and Sharing Results

Traditional evaluation of the success of work in health care usually involves measuring quality and safety outcomes, patient and staff satisfaction, identification of structure and process facilitators and barriers, and attainment of pre-defined goals. These measures of success hold true for evidence-based practice (EBP) work as well. However, the success of EBP work does not end at the conclusion of the project. In all aspects of the nursing organization, the use of evidence-based nursing practice findings must be valued and supported. EBP mentoring must highlight the importance of disseminating project results. Mentoring nurses to disseminate EBP findings is critical to ensure that these findings are made available to both providers and consumers of health care.

Considerable barriers to broad dissemination of EBP work exist. Organizations must develop capacity to support nurses in increasing their expertise in common strategies to ensure effective dissemination. This chapter focuses on common dissemination strategies that nurses can use both inside and outside the organization to share results of EBP projects.

Translation and Dissemination

Translation of evidence into practice can take a variety of paths and depends on the consistency or congruence of findings, the quantity of evidence, the strength and quality of studies, and other characteristics of the evidence that influence the advisability of implementing recommendations in the particular practice setting. Although translation and dissemination might seem like similar processes, differences between them exist. Translation includes decision making about what to do with the evidence and the subsequent implementation of the recommended plan of action. Dissemination is a translation technique that follows after the decision making and plan of action have been determined.

Merriam-Webster's online dictionary defines dissemination as to spread or disperse throughout (Merriam-Webster, 2009). With effective dissemination, organizations raise awareness and cultivate recognition that practice must be evaluated for change because of new evidence. The successful dissemination of the results of an EBP project is seen in the appropriate use of the new information and translation of the evidence into practice. However, effective dissemination involves a two-way communication process and is part of a well-developed strategy to regularly communicate results of EBP project work within the organization.

The National Center for the Dissemination of Disability Research (NCDDR) has identified 10 elements of an effective dissemination plan (NCDDR, 2001) to remind professionals of the importance of planning for dissemination from the start of proposal development to meet the challenge of timely dissemination (Table 10.1). This also applies to EBP project work. When a practice question is generated and the evidence search plan is developed, the EBP team should discuss strategies to communicate the results of the evidence search and who should be included in the dissemination plan.

Table 10.1: Ten Elements of an Effective Dissemination Plan (NCDDR, 2001)

1. **Goals:** Determine and document the goals of your dissemination effort for your proposed project.

2. **Objectives:** Associate each goal with one or more objectives that clarifies what you are trying to accomplish through your dissemination activities.

3. **Users:** Describe the scope and characteristics of the "potential users" that your dissemination activities are designed to reach for each of your objectives.

4. **Content:** Identify, at least, the basic elements of the projected content you have to disseminate to each of the potential user groups identified.

5. **Source(s):** Identify the primary source or sources that each potential user group is already tied into or most respects as an information source. Consider ways to partner with these sources in your dissemination efforts.

6. **Medium:** Describe the medium or media through which the content of your message can best be delivered to your potential users and describe the capabilities and resources that will be required of potential users to access the content for each medium to be used.

7. **Success:** Describe how you will know if your dissemination activities have been successful. If data is to be gathered, describe how, when, and who will gather it.

8. **Access:** Describe how you will promote access to your information and how you will archive information that may be requested at a later date. Consider that most people will use your project-related information when they perceive a need for it—not necessarily when you have completed your research project.

9. **Availability:** Identify strategies for promoting awareness of the availability of your research-based information and the availability of alternate available formats.

10. **Barriers:** Identify potential barriers that may interfere with the targeted users' access or utilization of your information and develop actions to reduce these barriers.

Reprinted with permission, National Institute on Disability and Rehabilitation Research (Project #H133A0311402, 2001), Retrieved December 30, 2009, from http://www.researchutilization.org/matrix/resources/dedp/

Internal Dissemination

The dissemination of EBP project results within the organization requires development of a communication strategy. This strategy includes the creation of several standard formats for communication of all EBP project work and a menu of individual strategies of potential relevance to a specific project. The most important question to answer when planning the communication strategy is "What's in it for me?" The staff must understand what the new evidence means for their everyday patient care and how the evidence can improve outcomes and quality of care. For example, if a new set of guidelines for care are developed and need to be implemented, share the highlights of the changes in practice with the staff (need-to-know versus nice-to-know) and emphasize how new testing recommendations or treatment changes can improve outcomes and quality of care provided.

Effective communication strategies consider how the information is disseminated, what format to use that is accessible to the majority of the staff, and how to make the evidence easy to read and use by busy staff. Organizations can use many venues for dissemination, such as newsletters, websites, bulletin boards, staff meetings, journal clubs, nursing grand rounds, orientation, and staff continuing education.

Newsletters

The use of an internal newsletter with an "EBP Column" is a nice regular opportunity to report on EBP projects. The newsletter should allow for a report of new practice questions, EBP teams forming that need additional members, EBP projects in progress, and finally, the results of EBP work completed. The dissemination of completed work should include plans for follow-up and translation so staff members see the work's value to their practice.

Websites

An EBP website is a valuable dissemination tool for the nursing department. A well-designed website includes the EBP model or approach used in the organization; appraisal tools and other important EBP resources; links to valuable EBP information outside of the organization, such as to the library, databases, and EBP educational sites; and a dedicated space for reporting on EBP projects, similar to the sections discussed previously for the newsletter. This space on the website can also serve as an archive for the history of EBP project work completed by nurses in the organization. Developing a standard tool for reporting on completed EBP work so that the nurses become familiar with a common format and know what to look for in the report of findings is also helpful.

Journal Clubs

A journal club is another great venue for dissemination of EBP information in the work environment. Most of us think of using a journal club for EBP work to discuss and appraise the evidence in a nonthreatening group format. However, organizations can also use it to review and disseminate new evidence or the results of an EBP project.

The important thing in developing a journal club is for the staff to have a good time and to actively participate in the discussion of the new evidence. Each unit or department must decide on the format for its own journal club, but be sure that the journal club is conducted in a way in which everyone feels comfortable. An interesting format for the busy nursing unit whose staff say they never have time to read the journal club article is a weekly journal club for a half hour that includes the reading of the article.

During the first week of the month, the article is distributed, and the group reads and discusses the abstract together. If the article is of interest, the group agrees to continue with the article the next week. If the article does not interest the group, another article is chosen and the reading cycle begins again. In the second week of the cycle, the group reads and discusses the introduction and discussion/conclusion of the article to understand the problem and quickly jump to what the authors found out in the study. During the third week, the group reads and discusses the literature review and the results. Finally, during the last weekly group meeting, the hardest section, the methods, is read and discussed. If this format works for you, keep the articles in a folder on the unit so that hard copies are available for each week. An unintended and positive consequence has been that staff members who are really interested in the article actually do read it prior to the next group meeting!

Continuing Education

You can perform continuing education outreach efforts to disseminate new evidence in a variety of ways. Oral presentations, such as nursing grand rounds, unit-specific educational meetings, and orientation, are excellent opportunities to present the latest results of an EBP project. Many EBP projects have broad appeal and applicability to many nurses in an organization; be prepared that your fellow nurses are going to be very interested in the project and how they might use the results in their clinical area. If you feel unprepared for this type of oral presentation, select a mentor from the nursing education department and work with that individual to develop your first presentation. Each time you present your work, it gets easier. Developing presentation skills within the organization can give the nurse valuable practice and confidence to make a successful presentation to an external audience.

Practice-Based Learning

Interdisciplinary, interactive practice-based learning where nurses, physicians, and other health professionals have the opportunity to discuss what the new evidence means for practice at the local level and for their individual patients facilitates buy-in and makes more likely a desired change in behavior. The educational offering should include discussion of the risks and benefits of the recommended new practice and how the new evidence or proposed change can fit with the organizational culture, provider practice preferences, nursing and other clinician expertise, and the local patient population.

Allow for discussion of differences in the local setting and, if they are significantly different from the setting in which the evidence was generated, what things are essential for the proposed translation. Likewise, discussion of facilitators and barriers to the change and lessons learned from previous translations are important to include in the education. Use the educational session as an opportunity to involve providers in generating the action plan for translation and let them plan how the new evidence can be translated into patient care.

Opinion Leaders

Use of respected opinion leaders in the organization can help to connect the new knowledge to the local context and increase buy-in and adoption of the proposed change in practice by other providers. Clinicians, in general, have concern about cookbook implementation of new evidence without proper discussion, feedback, and planning. Clinical expertise is important for deciding what and how evidence gets implemented into the new setting. Opinion leaders can offer sound advice and counsel.

Decision Support Systems

A strategy for dissemination that is gaining popularity is the use of decision support systems in health information technology. Decision support systems can be programmed to provide automated reminders, triggers, algorithms, and advice in the form of the new evidence at the point-of-care to aid in clinical decision making, to promote consistency of implementation, and to maintain standards. With these programmed reminders, nurses and other health care providers have regular encouragement to adopt the new evidence resulting in a positive change in practice.

Submitting an Application to the Institutional Review Board

The question of whether or not to submit an application to the Institutional Review Board (IRB) always comes up as the action plan is being developed, especially when the decision is made to conduct a rapid-cycle quality improvement study or a pilot study. The IRB is an administrative body established to protect the rights and welfare of human research subjects recruited to participate in research activities conducted under the auspices of the institution with which it is affiliated (Office for Human Research Protections, 1993). The first two questions the IRB asks are whether the activity involves research and whether it involves human subjects.

The Institutional Review Board Guidebook (Office for Human Research Protections, 1993) defines these two terms as follows:

- Research as "a systematic investigation, including research development, testing and evaluation, designed to develop or contribute to generalizable knowledge."

- Human subjects as "living individual(s) about whom an investigator (whether professional or student) conducting research obtains (1) data through intervention or interaction with the individual, or (2) identifiable private information."

According to the Institutional Review Board Guidebook, some subjects might be exempt from the regulations requiring IRB review, including those using educational testing and survey procedures where no identifying information is recorded that can link subjects to the data and where the disclosure of the data could not reasonably place the subjects at risk of civil or criminal liability or be damaging to the subjects' financial standing, employability, or reputation and research that involves the use of existing data, documents, or specimens, where no identifying information is recorded that can link subjects to the data (Office for Human Research Protections, 1993).

Research Versus Quality Improvement

At times your EBP team might find insufficient evidence to answer the practice question and decide to conduct a rapid-cycle quality improvement (QI) study or a pilot research study to fill that gap. "A clear understanding of the differentiation between QI and research will enhance evidence-based practice efforts that focus on improvement and strengthen studies intended to generate knowledge through research" (Newhouse, Pettit, Poe, & Rocco, 2006, p. 218). You should be careful to avoid misrepresenting quality improvement as research, the consequence of which can be poorly designed and interpreted studies, potential infringement on subject rights, or sanctions for noncompliance with federal or institutional policies. Conversely you can also face dangers in misrepresenting research as quality improvement in that ethical standards can be overlooked and human protections review can be bypassed. Consultation with the local IRB helps you to determine whether the planned activities fall under the quality improvement or research umbrella. Here is some helpful information to assist you to differentiate between quality improvement and research.

Research uses disciplined methods to answer questions or solve problems. Quality improvement uses specified methodologies to analyze current performance to improve quality of care and services.

Research activities are intended to generate new knowledge—knowledge that is intended to be generalized to a broader population of interest than the sample alone (Kring, 2008; Newhouse, Pettit, Poe, & Rocco, 2006). Quality improvement activities are aimed at internal process improvements—intended to benefit specific groups of patients (present and future) within the internal organization and are not intended to have any application outside the organization in which they are conducted (Newhouse et al., 2006; Kring, 2008). These activities are used as management tools to improve the care of specific patient populations within the organization or department in which the activities are conducted. You need to understand the distinction between quality improvement and research if your EBP team is considering conducting either type of inquiry for the action plan.

Research almost always involves some sort of risk to subjects, however minimal, and any benefits realized are usually to future patients or the scientific community that implements findings in the future (Kring, 2008). Quality improvement, on the other hand, rarely involves risk, and because only practices that have proven to be beneficial are tested, you see an anticipated benefit to current and future patients, staff, and providers in the particular organization or department.

If you are unsure about whether your EBP project action plan involving quality improvement or a pilot study should have IRB review, the safest road is to submit a query to your IRB for a consultation on the methods of the project. It is better to be safe than sorry at the conclusion of the project work.

External Dissemination

External dissemination of EBP findings involves presenting the result of your EBP project to the broader health care community to foster improved patient care and interdisciplinary collaboration. External dissemination usually involves three options: oral presentation, poster presentation, and written publication. External oral and poster presentations are usually peer reviewed and invited following the submission and review of an abstract. This section of the chapter focuses on the development of a successful abstract, poster, oral presentation, and manuscript.

Abstract

An abstract is a summary description of your work and must make sense as a stand-alone document. The abstract should describe the purpose, significance, and results of your work and what you recommend. It needs to answer the "so what?" question and describe succinctly what is new about your work and what you are adding to the current knowledge on the topic.

Types of Abstracts

Generally you have two types of abstracts. The first is a summary abstract that is submitted with a manuscript or grant proposal and provides a summary of what is to come in the submission. This abstract is written for a review committee. The second type of abstract is a conference abstract. This type of abstract is written for consideration to make an oral presentation or develop a poster for a professional or specialty organization meeting. The requirements for the abstract are usually described in a "Call for Abstracts" from the conference organizers. Watch for these announcements to be publicized many months before a meeting or convention either in the conference brochure or in a separate announcement. The conference abstract is written first for a review committee and second for the conference participants to whom you actually deliver your presentation or poster. The abstracts are often published in a conference overview booklet so that attendees can decide which sessions best meet their educational needs.

Word Limits, Objectives, and Keywords

Most abstracts have a word limit that can range from 100 to 500 words with 250 words being the most common. If you are submitting online, the text box is often designed to prevent you from exceeding the word limit. Be careful and use the word count feature to meet the guidelines as many reviews eliminate abstracts that go over the word limit.

If you are submitting an abstract to a conference, you often need to write two objectives for the presentation or poster session, and you might be asked to identify how your objectives meet the conference objectives or which conference objective the abstract is targeting. You might also be asked to provide "keywords" about your work. Keywords are often requested to determine how the abstract meets the conference goals or to assign the review of the abstract to a reviewer. In writing both the objectives and the keywords for the abstract, you are often determining whether, how, and by whom your abstract is going to be reviewed. Avoid writing in the first person, using "I" or "we," even though it was your project. Always write in third person for a formal submission. Careful attention to these additional steps in the process can help you to be successful.

Format

The format of the abstract depends on the person to whom you are submitting the abstract and the work itself. Pay close attention to the required format as outlined by the journal or the conference and include those words bolded as the topic area for each section. In that way, you can avoid leaving out an important part of the abstract and can show the reader that you have followed their format. However, most abstracts have similar essential sections:

1. **Problem statement or motivation for the work:** This section describes what question you are trying to answer or what problem you are trying to solve. It should also describe the scope and importance of the work, why people should care about the problem, and why it is going to be interesting to readers or conference attendees.

2. **Approach or methods:** This section describes what you did to get your results. For example, this would describe how you conducted your search, the evidence appraisal, and might also include important decisions you made in the approach to answering your question (for example, excluding international studies from the evidence search and review or limiting the search to English language or adults).

3. **Results:** The results section of the abstract tells the reader what you found or learned. It describes the answer to the question. With a limit to the number of words in most abstract submissions, how specific or general you are in this section depends on the magnitude of the results.

4. **Implications and recommendations:** This final section of the abstract describes the changes, if any, that should be implemented as a result of the work, whether the results are generalizable or specific, and what the next steps or future work might be.

The difference between a research and EBP abstract is the focus of each section. A research abstract includes more scientific methods and merits of the study, including research questions, hypotheses, statistical approaches, and limitations of the study. In contrast the EBP abstract focuses on the importance of the practice question for efficiency and effectiveness of practice, the appraisal of the current evidence, and discuss practice recommendations and innovations.

The successful abstract results in dissemination of the EBP project work in one of three formats: poster presentation, oral or podium presentation, or a publication. Figure 10.1 provides an example of a successful abstract submitted to the Doctor of Nursing Practice LLC Conference.

Title: Translating the Use of the 5A's Intervention to Improve Adult Type 2 Diabetes Self-Management

Goal: The 5A's behavioral intervention (ask, advise, agree, assists, and arrange) has been successfully used to improve behavioral risk factors in primary care. The purpose of this systematic review of the literature is to evaluate the evidence for use of the 5A's intervention to improve adult type 2 diabetes self-management by nurse practitioners in primary care.

Objectives: The participant will be able to

1. Evaluate the methodological quality of articles identified in the systematic review of the literature.

2. Review the strengths and limitations of the evidence for self-management interventions to improve glycemic control.

3. Determine whether the 5A's intervention is a feasible option to improve adult type 2 diabetes in primary care.

Summary: Although there is no identification of a "best practice" diabetic self-management intervention, there is clear evidence that overall interventions modestly improve glycemic control. Interventions that are patient-centered, intensive in nature, and in particular involve nurses or nurse practitioners are most effective. Nurse practitioner use of the 5A's intervention to improve adult type 2 diabetes self-management in primary care is a feasible option.

Figure 10.1: Successful Abstract Submitted to Doctor of Nursing Practice LLC Conference by Andrea Schram

Posters

Presenting a poster at a conference or convention usually results from the submission of an abstract as described previously to a "Call for Abstracts" from the conference organizers. You most often use posters to disseminate a work in progress, and presenting one affords several advantages. First, that sort of presentation is a great way to get comfortable with dissemination of your work without the pressure of a podium presentation. Second, it gives you the opportunity to interact and network with those in attendance during a poster presentation session and can allow for valuable feedback for the work that is still in progress. Preparation for a poster presentation involves more than the development of a great poster. It also means that you as the presenter need to discuss the main points of your work succinctly, aiming for less than one minute of interaction with conference attendees who are circulating in the poster session. To get their attention, you should have a sound bite to pique their interest, for example, a question to stimulate their curiosity in the topic (Have you ever wondered what the evidence is for doing…?).

Creating an effective poster is both an art and a science and requires careful planning and consideration to the message that you want to provide. The science involves the planning of format and message. The art involves the design of text, headings, color, and graphics.

The Science of Creating Posters

Posters are usually designed in two formats. The style you choose depends on the presentation venue, cost, and/or personal preference. The first format is a single-sheet format that is usually mounted on a corkboard in the conference room. The second format is a multipanel poster that is usually designed to sit on a table. Obviously, you need to find out what presentation venue is offered for the poster session before you begin the planning and development of your poster. You also need to consider portability of the poster to the conference. Can you carry the poster, can you put it in your luggage, or do you need a special case to pack the poster? It might be worth mailing/shipping the poster ahead of time to your hotel for ease and travel comfort. Check with the hotel about the proper procedure to insure that your poster is waiting for you on arrival.

The most important part of the development of the poster is the planning and organization of the poster message. Ask yourself a few questions to begin:

1. What is the message that I want to convey?

2. How do I want to convey the message?

3. What words/images/tables are critical to illustrate the message?

Keep the message simple, brief, and focused on the critical ideas. Determine what size poster you can have and create a life-size mockup of the poster with the main points. Remember to leave space across the top for a title and a list of authors and their employment site or site of the work. The sections of the poster should basically be the sections of the abstract you submitted. The methods section can be shortened or eliminated on the poster because most of those visiting your poster are going to be mainly interested in the results and your recommendations. You can provide a handout of the poster for conference attendees. Many poster handouts include a miniature of the poster on one side and then additional information or a copy of the abstract on the back. You can often gauge the interest in your work by the requests for handouts. Always have your business card available in case you run out of handouts so that attendees can e-mail you to request a copy of the handout.

After you have drafted the message of your poster, you need to edit for readability. Readability involves both format and flow of ideas. Limit the amount of text and stay focused on the message by using bulleted key points and begin to think about the design.

The Art of Creating Posters

The art of poster development is all about the design. Posters are designed left to right and top to bottom. The most important messages of your poster need to be visibly highlighted and positioned to catch the eye of those in attendance. If you design a poster with three columns, the most important messages should be at the top of the three columns. For example, the practice question should be on the upper left, the evidence summary can be displayed in the upper middle under the title, and the practice recommendations can be on the upper right-hand side of the poster display. Figure 10.2 illustrates the poster presentation.

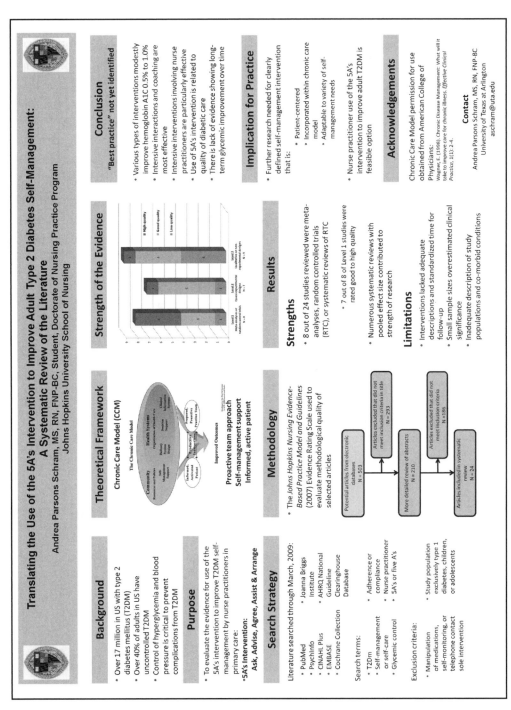

Figure 10.2: Successful Poster Presentation Submitted to Doctor of Nursing Practice LLC Conference by Andrea Schram

The use of headings, text, font, color, graphics, tables, charts, and pictures helps to communicate your planned message. Headings convey the major points of the message and help the attendee understand the project. Use only words that are absolutely necessary, evaluate the necessity of everything you place on the poster, and eliminate any redundancy or extraneous material. Vary the font to create a more visually pleasing poster with headings larger than subheadings and text to catch the eye. However, do not use more than three to four different fonts and use them consistently across sections of the poster. Never use less than a 12-point size font because of readability. Choose your colors for the poster carefully. Color borders, backgrounds, and contrasts are ways to add color to the poster but should be pleasing to the eye and not detract from the poster. Use graphics in the form of charts, tables, and pictures as much as possible to illustrate key points and substitute for text.

Several software packages, such as Microsoft PowerPoint, can help you to design the poster. See Table 10.2 for a quick guide to great websites for developing poster designs.

Table 10.2: Quick Guide to Poster Design Websites

1.   The Health Sciences Library of the New York Medical College has several very helpful websites for design of posters. The first website is a step-by-step guide on "How to Create a Poster Using PowerPoint" and the other two links are reference guides to Microsoft PowerPoint poster design: http://library.nymc.edu/access/create_PPposter.cfm   http://www.nymc.edu/Infotech/Site/Quick_References_Guide/powerpoint-quick-reference-2007.pdf   http://www.nymc.edu/Infotech/Site/Quick_References_Guide/powerpoint-quick-reference-2003.pdf
2.   The University of Washington has several public websites designed to assist in poster design: http://faculty.washington.edu/robinet/poster.html   http://sph.washington.edu/practicum/ppposter.asp

3. Colin Purrington from the Department of Biology at Swarthmore College in Pennsylvania has designed a very comprehensive website on designing scientific posters.

    http://www.swarthmore.edu/NatSci/cpurrin1/posteradvice.htm

4. The Teaching Learning and Technology Center at Texas Tech University has a very good poster tutorial with specific tips to increase success for poster creation and printing:

    http://www.tltc.ttu.edu/posters/How_to_Make_a_Poster_Using_Power-Point.pdf

5. The University of Kansas Medical Center has a general website on effective presentations (both oral and written) and it includes a link to creating posters:

    http://www.kumc.edu/SAH/OTEd/jradel/effective.html

Oral Presentation

An oral presentation is a great way to share expertise and the results of your EBP project work. However, many nurses do not like to make oral presentations. It has often been said that public speaking is one of the things people fear most, just ahead of death! To get over any barriers or fears to oral presentation, you can make a presentation in the work setting for practice and confidence before attempting an external oral presentation. In addition, you can use certain important strategies to increase your chances of delivering a winning oral presentation.

Preparation

Preparation is critical for the development and delivery of the presentation. The first preparation strategy is to know and understand your audience. Clarify the goals of the conference with the conference planners and assess if this is a specialty or multipurpose conference. This information can help you to determine the audience's knowledge level, experience, motivation, and understanding of the topic and assist you to develop the appropriate level of content for your presentation.

The next preparation strategy is to know what you want to accomplish. What is the goal of the presentation? Is the presentation designed to inform, persuade, and/or move the audience to action? In presenting results of an EBP project, you might want to accomplish each of these goals. You certainly want to provide the evidence that you have found and critiqued to the audience, and you might want to make recommendations for a practice change based on the evidence. You might also feel that you have to persuade the audience with the strength and quality of the evidence to change an approach to practice that has been embedded for a long time in tradition and ritual in their practice.

After you have determined the goal for the presentation, develop specific objectives. You might have submitted objectives when you submitted the abstract for review and acceptance to the conference. Revisit those objectives and add specific objectives for different sections of the presentation. These objectives can serve as an overall outline for the presentation.

The final stage of preparation is to develop the content and determine what you want to say to the audience. You should be able to state the "walk away" message in no more than one sentence. Select the appropriate resource material to use in the presentation and create a detailed outline to organize your material and begin content development. At this point, you have to decide what type of presentation aids you plan to use to get the message to the audience; for example, are you going to use a PowerPoint presentation, show a video, or develop a case study? Many professional meetings and conferences use PowerPoint as a visual aid for the presentations.

PowerPoint Tips

Here are a few basic tips for developing effective PowerPoint presentations:

1. Choose one design template for the entire presentation.

2. Limit the information on each slide.

3. Use the rule of "six," no more than six words on a line and no more than six lines on a slide.

4. Standardize the format, fonts, punctuation, capitalization, colors and contrast, and transitions and animation as much as possible.

5. Know the length of time for your presentation and develop no more than one slide per minute.

Writing the Script

After you have developed the content, write a script or text for the presentation. Give careful consideration to scripting your opening to the presentation to engage the audience and get their attention immediately. Common thought is that you only have 10 to 15 seconds to get their attention and to establish yourself as knowledgeable and worth listening to. The opening could include a direct statement of the significance of the EBP project to your unit or department. Tell the audience what led you on the journey to look for the evidence you are about to present. You could also use a more indirect approach by beginning your presentation with something of vital interest to the audience, a related important statistic, or a story or anecdote. After developing the main content, once again, give careful attention to the development of a powerful closing to your presentation. You should provide a summary of the main points and then challenge the audience, recommend a course of action or tell another story to drive home the message of your presentation. Always leave the audience with something to think about.

Other Considerations

Keep in mind these few final considerations for any type of presentation. First, practice is the key to any successful presentation. Be familiar with the content and do several practice runs to check timing and flow. Many peer-reviewed and invited oral presentations have a tight time limit, ranging from 20 minutes to 45 minutes. Often a moderator is assigned to the session to time the presentation and cue you when you have reached the time limit. You should be prepared to summarize your presentation if you have run out of time and have not finished.

Second, when you arrive at the conference, visit the assigned presentation room to view the floor plan seating arrangement of the room, the speaker accommodations (stage, podium, table, microphone, and so on), the presentation technology, and to assess how your presentation is going to be viewed. Be prepared that on the day of the presentation, the equipment might not work, and you still have to proceed. Never be so dependent on the equipment that you cannot continue and deliver your message. Many conferences have a "speaker-ready" room where you can view your PowerPoint on the conference's technology platform and take one more opportunity to practice your presentation and timing.

Appearance and rapport can affect the presentation delivery and should be considered when preparing for the presentation. Professional dress and a pleasant demeanor (open body language, smile, and eye contact) with the audience are essential to a successful delivery. Again, these things have to be learned and should be practiced. Even the most experienced speakers give consideration to dress and appearance at each presentation.

Finally, if you are involved in a team presentation, everyone should share the team focus and each team member should understand that their contribution is essential. Develop a master outline with time allocations for each team member, and attempt to match team members' expertise with their assigned topics. Decide ahead of time which team member is to coordinate the question and answer portion of the presentation.

Publication

If writing that article for publication sounds like something you don't think you could do, you are mistaken. Fear of writing is a similar barrier to dissemination as fear of public speaking. Your experience in EBP projects is very important work, and the profession needs to know about it. You can begin to write for publication in two simple ways. The first is to write with the team who were part of the EBP project and to develop the manuscript together. The second way is to find a mentor who has been successful with publishing and to work with that person on the manuscript. Either strategy can help you to jumpstart the writing process. Additionally, consider every abstract, poster, and oral presentation you do as the beginning of a manuscript for publication.

Authorship

The first issue to consider when developing a manuscript for publication is the matter of authorship. Some departments have developed their own detailed, written guidelines on authorship practices and make them available to everyone. Discuss these as you begin your work. If no formal guidelines exist, make sure that you discuss authorship prior to the onset of a working relationship and regularly so that people are comfortable asking questions about their work and how it is to be credited.

In 1978, a group of medical editors met in Vancouver, British Columbia, to establish guidelines for the format of manuscripts submitted to their journals. They became known as the Vancouver Group initially and are now called the International Committee of Medical Journal Editors (ICMJE). The requirements for manuscripts were first published in 1979; the latest version was developed in 2008 (ICMJE, 2008). According to the ICMJE's *Uniform Requirements for Manuscripts Submitted to Biomedical Journals: Writing and Editing for Biomedical Publication,* all persons designated as authors should qualify for authorship. Each author should have participated sufficiently in the work to take public responsibility for the content of the whole article. Authorship credit should be based on a potential author meeting all three of these criteria:

1. The potential author should make substantial contributions to conception and design, acquisition of data, or analysis and interpretation of data.

2. The potential author should participate in drafting the article or critically revising it for important intellectual content.

3. The potential author should give final approval of the version to be published.

Manuscript Development

So, how do you get started writing that article for publication? You have already decided that you want to publish your EBP project results. You have several publication options from which to choose: review of literature, an innovation report, a scientific report, a letter to the editor, and other journal-specific departments. Choose the publication option based on the significance of the content of the EBP project and the proposed readership. Next, you should select the journal to submit your manuscript. Review the author guidelines and to improve your chances for acceptance pay close attention to the required format for the manuscript preparation and for managing references and citations. Manuscripts that do not follow the prescribed guidelines are often returned to the author unreviewed. Prior to final selection of the journal, review the last 2 years of monthly indexes of the journal to make sure that it publishes the type of work you intend to submit and that no recent publication of similar work exists in that journal. You might also write a query letter to the editor of the journal to determine if interest in the manuscript topic exists.

A few tips can help you get started with the writing. First, develop an outline to help you organize the material and focus your content. Begin by developing major headings and then develop subheadings within each section. Make sure that you have researched the practice question thoroughly and review your records of any inclusion or exclusion decisions that you made during the evidence search process.

Format Options

You can use two types of outlines for scholarly writing. The first type of outline is the "IMRAD" or Introduction, Methods, Results, And Discussion format, which follows the process of scientific discovery. The ICMJE established this format for text of observational and experimental manuscripts submitted to biomedical journals. The Introduction section includes background on the study or project and answers the *why* question. You would also include a description of the problem in this section. The Methods section details the approach taken to study the problem and answers the questions of *when, where* and *how*? The Results section reports on the *what* question and discusses what was found. And the Discussion section explains what the results mean and discusses limitations and conclusions. Long articles might need subheadings within some sections (especially Results and Discussion) to clarify their content.

However, the ICMJE agrees that other article types, such as case reports, reviews, and editorials, probably need to be formatted differently (ICMJE, 2008). Unfortunately, scholarly accounts of the methods, experiences, and results of health care quality improvement work are often not published (Davidoff & Batalden, 2005). These improvement efforts focus primarily on making care better at local sites, but despite the local focus, improvement efforts frequently generate important new knowledge about systems of care and about how best to change those systems (Davidoff & Batalden, 2005). Davidoff and Batalden (2005) cite the many reasons for this failure to publish health care improvement work:

- Competing service responsibilities of and lack of academic rewards for improvement staff

- Editors' and peer reviewers' unfamiliarity with improvement goals and methods

- Lack of publication guidelines that are appropriate for rigorous, scholarly improvement work

They view this failure to publish as a serious deficiency, limiting the available evidence on efficacy, depriving staff of the opportunity and incentive to clarify thinking, slowing dissemination of established improvement work, inhibiting the discovery of innovations, and compromising the ethical obligation to return valuable information to the public.

A new outline format was developed and has reached a level of consensus as the format for reporting of improvement studies, Standards for Quality Improvement Reporting Excellence (SQUIRE) guidelines (see Figure 10.3). (Davidoff, Batalden, Stevens, Ogrinc & Mooney, 2008; Oermann, 2009). The SQUIRE outline format is also appropriate for reporting EBP project work and is being used in nursing journals. The SQUIRE basic outline format includes Introduction, Methods, Results, and Discussion, but the suggested subheadings under each section allow for report of more relevant information to improvement work including information about the planned intervention, the context in which the intervention will be implemented, and effectiveness evaluation (Davidoff et al., 2008). See Figure 10.3 for a complete description of the SQUIRE Guidelines.

SQUIRE Guidelines
(Standards for QUality Improvement Reporting Excellence)
Final revision – 4-29-08

- These guidelines provide a framework for reporting formal, planned studies designed to assess the nature and effectiveness of interventions to improve the quality and safety of care.

- It may not be possible to include information about every numbered guideline item in reports of original formal studies, but authors should at least consider every item in writing their reports.

- Although each major section (i.e., Introduction, Methods, Results, and Discussion) of a published original study generally contains some information about the numbered items within that section, information about items from one section (for example, the Introduction) is often also needed in other sections (for example, the Discussion).

Text section; Item number and name	Section or Item description
Title and abstract	*Did you provide clear and accurate information for finding, indexing, and scanning your paper?*
1. Title	a. Indicates the article concerns the improvement of quality (broadly defined to include the safety, effectiveness, patient-centeredness, timeliness, efficiency, and equity of care) b. States the specific aim of the intervention c. Specifies the study method used (for example, "A qualitative study," or "A randomized cluster trial")
2. Abstract	Summarizes precisely all key information from various sections of the text using the abstract format of the intended publication
Introduction	*Why did you start?*
3. Background Knowledge	Provides a brief, non-selective summary of current knowledge of the care problem being addressed, and characteristics of organizations in which it occurs
4. Local problem	Describes the nature and severity of the specific local problem or system dysfunction that was addressed
5. Intended improvement	a. Describes the specific aim (changes/improvements in care processes and patient outcomes) of the proposed intervention b. Specifies who (champions, supporters) and what (events, observations) triggered the decision to make changes, and why now (timing)
6. Study question	States precisely the primary improvement-related question and any secondary questions that the study of the intervention was designed to answer
Methods	*What did you do?*
7. Ethical issues	Describes ethical aspects of implementing and studying the improvement, such as privacy concerns, protection of participants' physical well-being, and potential author conflicts of interest, and how ethical concerns were addressed
8. Setting	Specifies how elements of the local care environment considered most likely to influence change/improvement in the involved site or sites were identified and characterized
9. Planning the intervention	a. Describes the intervention and its component parts in sufficient detail that others could reproduce it b. Indicates main factors that contributed to choice of the specific intervention (for example, analysis of causes of dysfunction; matching relevant improvement experience of others with the local situation)

SQUIRE Publication Guidelines – Final revision – 4-29-08
Page 2

Text section; Item number and name	Section or Item description
Planning the intervention (continued)	c. Outlines initial plans for how the intervention was to be implemented: e.g., *what* was to be done (initial steps; functions to be accomplished by those steps; how tests of change would be used to modify intervention), and *by whom* (intended roles, qualifications, and training of staff)
10. Planning the study of the intervention	a. Outlines plans for assessing how well the intervention was implemented (dose or intensity of exposure) b. Describes mechanisms by which intervention components were expected to cause changes, and plans for testing whether those mechanisms were effective c. Identifies the study design (for example, observational, quasi-experimental, experimental) chosen for measuring impact of the intervention on primary and secondary outcomes, if applicable d. Explains plans for implementing essential aspects of the chosen study design, as described in publication guidelines for specific designs, if applicable (see, for example, www.equator-network.org) e. Describes aspects of the study design that specifically concerned internal validity (integrity of the data) and external validity (generalizability)
11. Methods of evaluation	a. Describes instruments and procedures (qualitative, quantitative, or mixed) used to assess a) the effectiveness of implementation, b) the contributions of intervention components and context factors to effectiveness of the intervention, and c) primary and secondary outcomes b. Reports efforts to validate and test reliability of assessment instruments c. Explains methods used to assure data quality and adequacy (for example, blinding; repeating measurements and data extraction; training in data collection; collection of sufficient baseline measurements)
12. Analysis	a. Provides details of qualitative and quantitative (statistical) methods used to draw inferences from the data b. Aligns unit of analysis with level at which the intervention was implemented, if applicable c. Specifies degree of variability expected in implementation, change expected in primary outcome (effect size), and ability of study design (including size) to detect such effects d. Describes analytic methods used to demonstrate effects of time as a variable (for example, statistical process control)
Results	*What did you find?*

13. Outcomes	a) Nature of setting and improvement intervention
	    i. Characterizes relevant elements of setting or settings (for example, geography, physical resources, organizational culture, history of change efforts), and structures and patterns of care (for example, staffing, leadership) that provided context for the intervention
	    ii. Explains the actual course of the intervention (for example, sequence of steps, events or phases; type and number of participants at key points), preferably using a time-line diagram or flow chart
	    iii. Documents degree of success in implementing intervention components
	    iv. Describes how and why the initial plan evolved, and the most important lessons learned from that evolution, particularly the effects of internal feedback from tests of change (reflexiveness)
	b) Changes in processes of care and patient outcomes associated with the intervention
	    i. Presents data on changes observed in the care delivery process
	    ii. Presents data on changes observed in measures of patient outcome (for example, morbidity, mortality, function, patient/staff satisfaction, service utilization, cost, care disparities)

SQUIRE Publication Guidelines – Final revision – 4-29-08
Page 3

Text section; Item number and name	Section or Item description
Outcomes (continued)	iii. Considers benefits, harms, unexpected results, problems, failures iv. Presents evidence regarding the strength of association between observed changes/improvements and intervention components/context factors v. Includes summary of missing data for intervention and outcomes
Discussion	*What do the findings mean?*
14. Summary	a. Summarizes the most important successes and difficulties in implementing intervention components, and main changes observed in care delivery and clinical outcomes b. Highlights the study's particular strengths
15. Relation to other evidence	Compares and contrasts study results with relevant findings of others, drawing on broad review of the literature; use of a summary table may be helpful in building on existing evidence
16. Limitations	a. Considers possible sources of confounding, bias, or imprecision in design, measurement, and analysis that might have affected study outcomes (internal validity) b. Explores factors that could affect generalizability (external validity), for example: representativeness of participants; effectiveness of implementation; dose-response effects; features of local care setting c. Addresses likelihood that observed gains may weaken over time, and describes plans, if any, for monitoring and maintaining improvement; explicitly states if such planning was not done d. Reviews efforts made to minimize and adjust for study limitations e. Assesses the effect of study limitations on interpretation and application of results
17. Interpretation	a. Explores possible reasons for differences between observed and expected outcomes b. Draws inferences consistent with the strength of the data about causal mechanisms and size of observed changes, paying particular attention to components of the intervention and context factors that helped determine the intervention's effectiveness (or lack thereof), and types of settings in which this intervention is most likely to be effective c. Suggests steps that might be modified to improve future performance d. Reviews issues of opportunity cost and actual financial cost of the intervention
18. Conclusions	a. Considers overall practical usefulness of the intervention b. Suggests implications of this report for further studies of improvement interventions
Other information	*Were other factors relevant to conduct and interpretation of the study?*
19. Funding	Describes funding sources, if any, and role of funding organization in design, implementation, interpretation, and publication of study

Figure 10.3: The SQUIRE Guidelines, with extensive additional resources, is available free from http://www.squire-statement.org/

You can use either of the two outline formats for manuscript preparation for EBP project work, and a combination of the two could be useful. Using the PET (Practice question, Evidence, Translation) process as an outline format with an

Introduction and Discussion section also makes sense. To start the manuscript writing, begin with the development of the Introduction, which includes the goal of the EBP project, a background discussion of the problem, the current status, and why the problem is important.

The second section of the manuscript, the Practice Question, includes a statement of the practice question and a discussion of the scope of the project work, including development of the project management plan with timeline and assignment of responsibilities. This discussion of who does what, when, and how gives the reader a feel for the development of the work.

The third section of the manuscript, the Evidence section, provides a report of the logical sequence of the search for evidence. It includes a list of the search terms, search strategies, databases used, and any inclusion and exclusion criteria developed. This section also includes a discussion of how the review was conducted, by whom, what tools were used for the appraisal of strength and quality of evidence, and how the evidence was summarized. Finally, this section should make a statement on the strength of the evidence and discuss practice recommendations based on the strength of the evidence.

The fourth section of the EBP project manuscript is the Translation section. Here you discuss the implementation plan, including practice changes if sufficient evidence strength exists, or discuss the design and results of the pilot study. If the pilot is successful, you present strategies for a full implementation and dissemination of findings, including the communication plan to share the results of the work. The final section of the EBP manuscript is the Discussion and Conclusions of the work, including lessons learned, final recommendations, and a discussion of what comes next.

Summary

Embracing the concept of EBP is easy, but implementing it in practice presents many challenges (Oermann, 2008). One of the greatest of those challenges is the translation and dissemination of the results of EBP projects both inside and outside of the organization. The importance of direct involvement of front-line staff first in leading EBP projects and then in disseminating the results of those projects cannot be overemphasized (Burns, Dudjak, & Greenhouse, 2009). The dissemination strategy for EBP project results must be two-pronged and must include a communication strategy for inside the organization and the three Ps of dissemination (posters, presentations, and publications) for external communication. Only through a comprehensive approach to translation and sharing of the results of EBP work can the profession move from tradition and ritual to a practice based on a spirit of inquiry that searches for the most current and relevant evidence for each practice setting.

References

Burns, H. K., Dudjak, L., & Greenhouse, P. K. (2009). Building an evidence-based practice infrastructure and culture: A model for rural and community hospitals. *Journal of Nursing Administration, 39*(7/8), pp. 321–325.

Davidoff, F., & Batalden, P. (2005). Toward stronger evidence on quality improvement. Draft publication guidelines: The beginning of a consensus project. *Quality and Safety in Health Care, 14*, pp. 319–25.

Davidoff F, Batalden P, Stevens D, Ogrinc G, Mooney S. (2008). Publication guidelines for quality improvement in health care: Evolution of the SQUIRE project. Qual Saf Health Care 2008;17[Supplement 1]:i3-i9.

International Committee for Medical Journal Editors. (2008). Uniform requirements for manuscripts submitted to biomedical journals: Writing and editing for biomedical publication. Retrieved December 20, 2009, from http://www.icmje.org/

Johns Hopkins Medicine Institutional Review Board. (2007). *Table 10.2 Johns Hopkins Medicine Organizational Policy on Quality Improvement/Quality Assurance Activity 102.2(a)*. Retrieved December 20, 2009, from http://irb.jhmi.edu/Policies/102_2a.html

Kring, D.L. (2008). Research and quality improvement: Different processes, different evidence. *MedSurgNursing, 17* (3), pp. 162-169.

Merriam-Webster. (2009). *Merriam-Webster Online Dictionary.* Retrieved December 20, 2009, from www.merriam-webster.com/dictionary/dissemination.

National Institute on Disability and Rehabilitation Research (Project #H133A0311402, 2001), Retrieved December 30, 2009, from http://www.researchutilization.org/matrix/resources/dedp/

Newhouse, R. P., Pettit, J. C., Poe, S., & Rocco, L. (2006). The slippery slope: Differentiating between quality improvement and research. *Journal of Nursing Administration, 36(4)*, pp. 211–219.

Oermann, M. (2009). SQUIRE guidelines for reporting improvement studies in healthcare: Implications for nursing publications. *Journal of Nursing Care Quality, 24(2)*, pp. 91–5.

Office for Human Research Protections. (1993). *Institutional Review Board guidebook.* Retrieved December 28, 2009, from http://www.hhs.gov/ohrp/irb/irb_chapter1.htm

SQUIRE. (2009). SQUIRE Standards for Quality Improvement Reporting Excellence. Retrieved December 31, 2009, from http://squire-statement.org/guidelines/

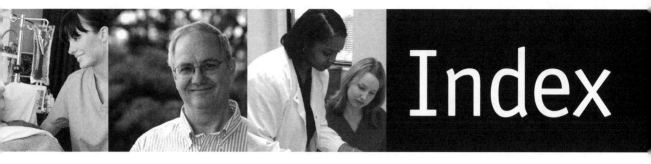

Index

D

E

F

J

N

O

P

S

T

V

W–Z

U

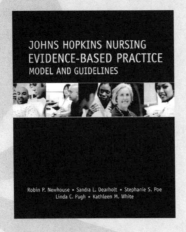
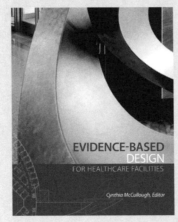
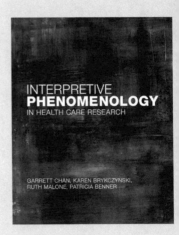
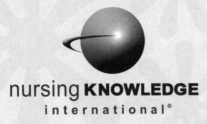